The War On Sleep

How it started
How we lost
How you can recover

By Michael Voss

ISBN Number: 978-0-578-17602-4

Printed in the United States of America

First Edition September 2020

For the millions of people who think they are sleeping fine, but who in reality are not, and the millions of others who know they are not sleeping well. Soon, you will all know the life-changing joy of good sleep.

Contents

Section 1: Background and Preparation

"Strategy without tactics is the slowest route to victory.
Tactics without strategy is the noise before defeat. "

-Sun Tzu

Disclaimer: Read This First

What you are about to read is the culmination of over a decade of my personal research and experimentation. Sometimes my experiments and observations were accidental, other times they were thoroughly planned and scientifically executed. The consistent factor is that they were always performed with one thing in mind: getting a better night's sleep. My secondary objective was to never damage my health and, whenever possible, to improve it. Fortunately, I discovered that improving one's health goes hand in hand with improving one's sleep, and I encountered few if any downsides.

It is important that you read this book fully understanding that, while I do not consider myself much different from many other people whose sleep could use improvement, no two people are quite the same when it comes to sleep. Some things that work for me may not work for you and some things that didn't help me at all may work like magic for you. It is my hope that I can impart to you the overall understanding I have developed of the sleep process so that you can make informed decisions that will lead you to the most optimal outcome. I do not intend to give you a fish, instead I intend to teach you how to fish for yourself.

Because sleep is a critical component of health, it is imperative that you be screened by a physician and, preferably, one who is a sleep specialist before making any radical changes to your lifestyle, habits, or medications. Some of the things described in this book cannot be obtained without the assistance of a physician anyway so, at some point, you may need to consult one. Something worth bearing in mind when searching for a doctor is that there is wide variability in the quality of physicians and sleep specialists, so you may want to read this book entirely before setting about finding one.

Do not let this disclaimer scare you off; much of the time during which I was doing my research, I did not have assistance from physicians nor the benefit of health insurance. The conditions under which I evaluated my own health and sleep were not always optimal. However, they were what I had at the time and I made due. You can, too. If I've done my job, this book should provide you with better tools and a starting place much further along the path to good sleep.

My original intent was not to write a book nor to share my findings in any way. I was only trying to resolve my own terrible sleep issues. However, after improving my own sleep, I became attuned to the deep suffering of people around me and noticed that not only were they in dire straits, they didn't have the tools to get out of the mess they were in. Whenever I bring up the subject of sleep and discuss my experiences, people are always eager to ask questions and learn more. In my 15+ years of research, it has become obvious to me that sleep deprivation is nothing less than an epidemic (indeed, in the intervening period, the US Centers for Disease Control have made that exact declaration) and this book is my attempt to put an end to it. It is my sincere belief that sleep disorders are underlying our national epidemics of obesity, diabetes, stroke, heart disease, cancers, and shortened lifespan, ailments which have only come to be leading causes of death in the past 120 years or so. I have greatly improved my own life, and I hope that I can do the same for the millions of people out there by sharing what I have learned to avert a current or future health disaster.

With that said, please be careful and take all reasonable precautions when following any of the advice in this book. I have done my best to always give accurate supporting information and, wherever possible, I have quoted research, facts, sources and statistics. Where I have described my own experiences, I have also been careful to be as accurate as possible. I am not a physician, and your health is the most valuable thing you possess, so it is your responsibility to take all reasonable precautions and consult with a physician before following any advice in this book or if you experience any adverse effect at any time.

Now, with that out of the way, let's find out how the War on Sleep got started, and how we can put an end to it.

Preface

One of the wisest people I have ever known once said that no good thing happens quickly. I have come to find this to be very true.

The work you are about to read has taken me nearly 15 years to complete. My research and experimentation are ongoing and many times I was sure I had gotten to a point where I needed to get what I'd learned out into the world, only to hit a new obstacle that had to be solved. Other times, science would crack yet another of the mysteries of sleep in a way that needed to be included. Or, perhaps I'd find I needed more data to really determine for certain what I had observed in some instance. Never in my life have I put so much time and effort into any one thing, and it has been worth every minute.

When I first began to try to solve the puzzle of sleep for myself, it was becoming a life and death need for me, although I may not have known it at the time. It was during the run up to the Great Recession of 2008 when the world was an uncertain, frightening place. Compounding the loss of income and wealth I had suddenly suffered, like many others, I had long been suffering from major depressive disorder accompanied (as it generally always is) by terrible sleep disturbances. Climbing out of that deep chasm was a long, arduous process and many times along the way I thought I was ready to complete this book, but I wasn't. As I came to learn, nothing good happens fast.

Today we find ourselves, once again, in a devastating and uncertain time as COVID-19 rages across the globe like wildfire causing the greatest disruption to human life that I have ever seen. As I absorb the daily updates and wonder when life will get back to anything resembling normal, I have realized two important things: the first is that all I have learned about sleep is the most valuable thing I have. I sleep every night since this crisis began at literally the best levels ever despite some of the worst conditions I have ever seen. Secondly, I have realized that NOW is the time to share all I know with everyone I can as quickly as possible. There will never be a time when being able to sleep well will be more difficult and of greater value to more people, so I have dropped everything to do final assembly of all I have learned and get it out to all who can benefit from it.

The COVID-19 pandemic has served as a sort of a final test for me. While the quarantine and shutdown of most things sounds idyllic for better sleep on the surface, far more people are having trouble sleeping due to the offsetting worry about their loved ones, jobs, income, homes, and everything else that is suddenly at risk. While I cannot cure the current or future issues that will affect us all, I can help you to sleep well no matter what the future may hold.

Michael Voss
Los Angeles
2020

Why I Wrote This Book and Why You Should Read It

When I start reading any new book, I want to know two things as quickly as possible: 1) Does the author actually have anything valuable to tell me? and 2) What is it? I don't want to waste a minute reading something that has no valuable information for me. There are countless articles, books, and sources of all kinds out there every day professing to tell you how to sleep better. Some of them are useful and others are nothing more than recycled, outdated collections of clichés that will not really help anyone much. Others are things which are actually wrong or misinterpreted and will make your sleep worse. So, how do you determine what is of value and why should you listen to what I have to say? Well, because I have spent 15 years working on a solution to the problem of sleep, and I can now demonstrate dramatic results. In short, I can put my money where my mouth is and show you proof of what I have accomplished, so I will start by doing so.

Over the last 6 or 7 years, devices and programs to graphically track sleep quality (with accuracy rivaling some medical sleep study labs) have become available, and I have used many of them. To date, I have over 2000 nights' worth of my sleep data recorded and, as you can see in the upcoming graphs

, in the past 6 years my sleep quality has improved from around 60% to 90% and climbing. I do not present speculative or idle advice in these pages; everything I relate I have tested personally and documented. The raw data is available to anyone wishing to see it on the website waronsleep.com. The information on my sleep which you see just ahead and throughout this book was collected with an excellent free app for IOS and Android called Sleep Cycle™ - more on that a bit later. You may notice some changes in the appearance of the Sleep Cycle graphics from different points in time as it's interface and appearance has evolved quite a bit over 6+ years that I have used it, but the information is unchanged.

How to Get Maximum Benefit from This Book

I have divided this book into four general sections. First is a short section detailing how my sleep has improved over the last 6 years and how it compares to the rest of the world – my credentials so that you know I speak credibly. After this are three major sections comprising the rest of the book. The first is a history and explanation of how we, as a society, got into trouble with sleep over the past 100+ years. The second is an in-depth description of the problem as it exists and affects most of us today. The last section is a detailed explanation of how to track your sleep starting immediately along with detailed information about the many things I have tested and now use regularly to significantly improve my sleep so that you can apply them as well and gauge your improvement.

I strongly encourage you to read this book from start to finish (though not necessarily at once, just in order) because there is a very big picture to how we have come to have culturally bad sleep habits and once you understand it as a whole you will be much better able to adapt and overcome the obstacles to good sleep as I have. It is a huge advantage to understand the big picture. I am not giving you some simple medicine or trick for one good night's sleep tonight – I intend to help you understand an entire society gone wrong, how it happened, and how to get back to normal as I have.

Please resist any temptation to read ahead and read and absorb all you can in detail in the written sequence. I promise you will benefit from it very soon.

My Sleep Quality Over the Last 6 Years

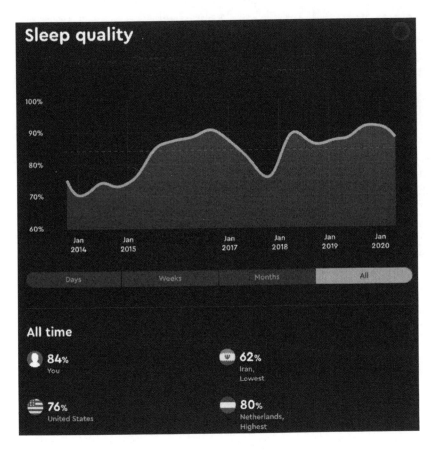

My average sleep quality (measured by the excellent free app Sleep Cycle) over the past 6 years has improved from under 60% to over 90%. The above graph loses the furthest outlying data points, but my lowest sleep quality was around 57% and I have had many nights at 100%. Take note of that dip in mid-2017; that was one of those detours that slowed the completion of this book and I will get into that a bit later. To get a better idea of how my sleep looks today, let's look at the last 6 months:

My Sleep Quality Over the Last 6 Months

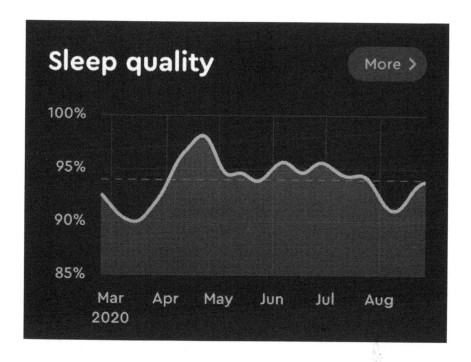

The above graph shows my sleep during the last 6 months, which just happens to also be the duration of the COVID-19 pandemic so far. The dip in March is when the pandemic hit. The subsequent spike was from my focusing on sleep even more than usual and being determined to not let the pandemic compound problems by affecting my sleep. The result has been that, even during the pandemic, I have slept extremely well and recorded some of my highest sleep quality levels in the entire 2000 nights since I began collecting data.

You can also see that it is rare for my sleep quality to dip below 90%. While making final revisions to this book, I logged 7 consecutive nights at 100% sleep quality during the pandemic- a personal record for me. The COVID-19 pandemic has been a sort of final exam for me, and I think it is an understatement to say I have passed. I have all the same worries, fears and concerns as everyone else around the world, but I have the distinct advantage that I am sleeping well every night.

A Terrible Night's Sleep From 6 Years Ago

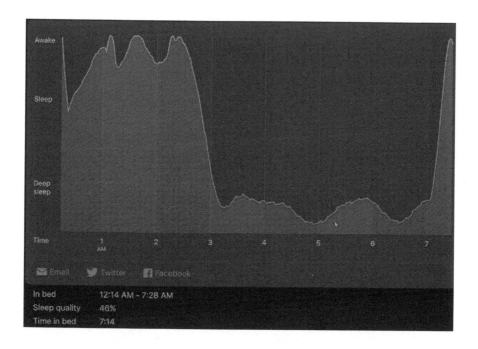

This is one of the worst nights of sleep I ever recorded from 2014 when I first started keeping records. Despite being in bed for over 7 hours, I only actually slept somewhere over 4 hours. If you have ever awakened feeling like you were run over by a truck and mentally barely able to even think, that's what a night like this translates to in the morning. Over the past 6 years, I have come to find any night under about 85% sleep quality to be unacceptable for me.

A Recent Excellent Night's Sleep

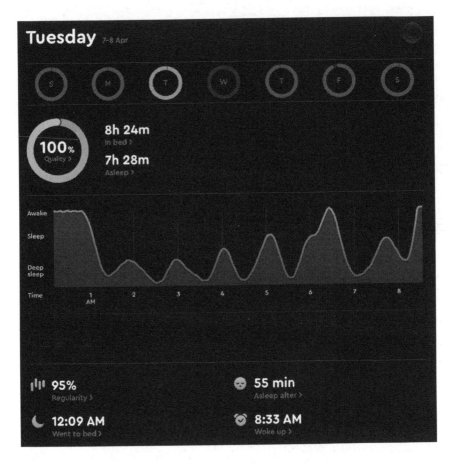

One of many more recent good nights where my sleep quality was 100%. Notice that I slept through the whole night with a normal, repeating 90-minute cycle between deeper and shallower phases of sleep. I also awakened slightly early at around 6:30AM but simply went back to sleep until I had a full and proper night's sleep. I have trained myself to do this over time and will tell you how to do so as well.

As you can see, the improvement I have made is dramatic, consistent, and still ongoing, even after over 6 years. Interestingly, the makers of Sleep Cycle began collecting data from users willing to voluntarily (and anonymously) submit it over the past 5 years or so. While it changes a bit from day to day, generally one country or another remain in the top and bottom spots for significant periods of time. Japan consistently had the worst average sleep quality at around 60% (This is absolutely horrible! I can tell you from having had nights of that quality.) until around April of 2015. At that time, Saudi Arabia became the worst sleeping country with national average sleep quality scores in the low 60 percentage and has remained there very consistently. It is interesting to note that almost to the week when Saudi Arabia moved into this spot, the Tesla Model 3 electric vehicle was announced and began taking orders worldwide selling over 200,000 pre-orders in about a week. Prior to this, during the preceding 2 years or so, the United States became the world's number one oil producer and Saudi Arabian citizens began having to pay taxes for the first time ever, began paying far more for gasoline, and were no longer eligible for cushy, state subsidized jobs as they have been for decades. It is a telling statistic that I actually anticipated happening, but I never guessed it would have such near exact timing. Saudi Arabia has since dominated the bottom spot for the most part. I don't know if they are aware of it, but our intelligence agencies could learn much from utilization of global sleep data.

The Netherlands and New Zealand, by contrast, often have the highest sleep quality of any country. I do not know the reasons for this, but it is something I intend to look into in the future. During the week of April 15th of this year, just after the Pandemic hit and I focused on prioritizing my sleep even more than usual, I had an average sleep quality score of 98% giving me literally one of the best sleep quality score averages in the world - in the top 2%. This was 17% higher than the highest national average in New Zealand, 23% higher than the US average, and 35% higher than the lowest average in Saudi Arabia.

My Sleep Quality Compared to the World the Week of April 15th, 2020

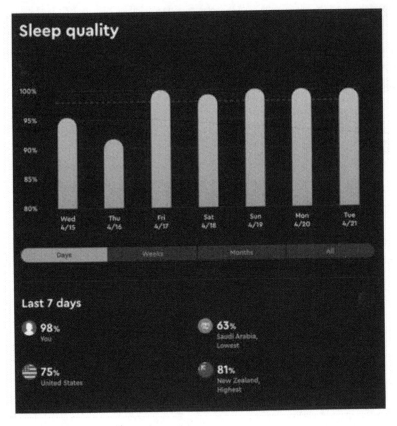

I sleep better than most of the people on Earth now.

One thing is immediately clear from all of these charts: I have cracked the code to getting consistently good sleep. After seeing my stellar sleep turnaround, if you find yourself pining for deep, restful, restorative sleep, such as I have achieved, the best thing you can do is continue reading and get ready to learn some things and make some changes.

Why Most Sleep Improvement Books Are Not Helpful and Why This One Is Different

There are an ever-increasing number of books available today on the subject of sleep improvement. Clearly, the long-neglected problem is now finally being recognized and many people are trying to address it. So, why aren't we all reading these books and sleeping better?

The answer is simple and only after my decade plus journey to fix my own sleep is it now clear to me: the reason most sleep solutions don't work for all people is because there are many different causes of poor sleep. While they fall under some general cause categories, some things will work for many people, but many things will only work for people with specific issues and will do nothing for the others. It is a mistake to throw general solutions at a multi-faceted problem without first collecting data and looking closely at the specific problem before attempting to rectify it.

Sometimes, inspirations for problem-solving appear out of the blue. Many of you will know Joe Rogan, a comedian who has an excellent podcast which I have listened to for years. Joe is a guy of above average intelligence, well spoken, and generally very pragmatic and scientific in his approach to things. He is, to large degree, a biohacker, as many of my friends and I consider ourselves to be. If you know who Tim Ferriss is, you already have a pretty good idea of what a biohacker generally is. A biohacker for the unfamiliar is a citizen scientist of sorts who focuses on things generally related to improving human biology. Athletic performance improvement, sleep improvement, and extending longevity are the specific areas I have been interested and working in informally for over 20 years now. Many of the things I and other biohackers first experimented with 20+ years ago, such as testosterone replacement therapy, are accepted common therapies today. Many of us started doing these things long before they were even contemplated by mainstream medicine. We have long looked upon ourselves as test pilots and willing barrier breakers and my personal belief is that we have done immeasurable good. Others may have different opinions, but I believe the test of time has strongly supported my belief about the efficacy and benefits of biohacking and I think in the future it will continue to gain momentum at an ever-increasing pace.

Years ago, I heard Joe discuss how he resolved his sleep problems by seeing a dentist who made him a custom mouthpiece which prevented him from snoring and effectively cured his sleep issues. Sometime later, I recalled this information and looked up the dentist after suddenly developing a similar issue with snoring, which I discuss in detail later. This dentist was very expensive, and did a fair amount of analytical work to provide a custom appliance for me – a mouthpiece which made things tremendously worse. In fact, it was so bulky it caused me to gag at times, but I was willing to train myself to sleep with it if it would work for me. It didn't, and I ended up throwing the $3000 device in the trash and never seeing the dentist again. Sometime after this, I discovered why the device had not worked and how the dentist had entirely failed to diagnose the cause of my snoring properly, despite the fact that it would have been easily done. He had tried to apply a one-size-fits-all solution to me, and it did not work. There is a well-worn old saying: If all you have is a hammer, every problem looks like a nail. Joe Rogan believed that the device which solved his issue (his tongue obstructing his airway) would work for all others and recommended it as such for others who snore. In someone like me, who had a completely different reason for snoring, it was totally ineffective and even rather dangerous. The problem isn't that he wasn't giving helpful information – for some people he was – the problem was that he was not aware that he was recommending a treatment for one very specific type of airway obstruction that causes snoring in some people when there are *many* other types of such obstructions that can make one snore. It helped him, so he thought it would help everyone and wanted to share it. Unfortunately, in some cases, such advice can do more harm than good.

Another similar thing recently occurred, coincidentally enough, when Elon Musk made an appearance on... Joe Rogan's podcast. Musk, another person for who I have immense respect, expressed an opinion that eating before sleep is terrible for anyone and then went into a discussion of how food and alcohol before sleep affect (without specifically segregating out) persons suffering from Acid Reflux disease or GERD, once again dispensing advice for all which would not affect those unaffected by these issues. As I have suffered from Acid Reflux for around 20 years now and take medication for it daily, I am *keenly* aware that if I were to eat or consume alcohol or certain foods close to bed time without having taken my medication it would be a VERY uncomfortable outcome which would disturb my sleep significantly. However, since I take my medication daily, I can eat and drink right up to bedtime, including moderate alcohol, with no issue. Once again, offering individually relevant medical advice to a large audience as if it were a cure-all when, in truth, it may only be applicable to a small subset of that audience could cause someone to take a wrong turn in improving their sleep.

While Joe's advice would help those with a similar tongue obstruction and Elon's is of value for those suffering from untreated GERD, the majority of people would not benefit from these solutions. People with scientific mindsets should know better than to make such untested, general recommendations based on little or no collected data (for themselves or others they are sharing it with), but they are just trying to help. We are in the early days of the War on Sleep, and this is what is known as the 'fog of war'.

Many such people want similarly to help others in their quest for better sleep by sharing what has helped them, but in a lot of cases it would be better if they said nothing at all since they are not presenting a complete picture which will help the greatest number of people. That is what I shall endeavor to do in the pages ahead.

Introduction

"The key to growth is the introduction of higher dimensions of consciousness into our awareness."

-Lao Tzu

How Did You Sleep Last Night?

When I talk to people about sleep, individually or in groups, this is usually the first thing I ask them. Frequently, one or several people tell me, very confidently, that they slept "great". (It is interesting to note that the two most common answers I get are great and terrible – not much in between.) My next question usually is, "Really? How do you *know*?" They generally now either stop and think, possibly for the first time ever, how DO they really know how they slept or, more often, they just launch into a series of long-held beliefs about why they *must* be sleeping well – usually with the false confidence of someone well versed in protecting long-held, dogmatic beliefs in something they really have no data on.

Something I learned (relatively) early in life is that there is a DISTINCT difference between what a person KNOWS and what they BELIEVE. Most people I talk to BELIEVE they slept well, just about none of them KNOW that. By contrast, I KNOW how I slept last night, and I can tell you pretty precisely and support that with actual hard data – graphically and in great detail as you have seen.

The fact of the matter is that, when you are sleeping, you are *unconscious*, so you really have no idea as to what is going on either at that time or anytime later. *None*. If you were in a court of law, you could not bear witness as to anything that occurred during that time. You literally do not know. If you did, we wouldn't have sleep study labs staffed by doctors and set up with stacks of cutting-edge scientific equipment to evaluate people's sleep – the doctor would just ask them how they slept and save a lot of trouble and expense! Most people rely on what empirical evidence they can gather upon waking: You know you went to bed at 11:30 and woke up at 7:30; you don't recall waking up, recall a bit of a dream, and you're not tired, so it must have been a good night's sleep, right? Not necessarily. Maybe you slept 9 hours because you stopped breathing 80 times per hour and could never get sufficient restful sleep that you would have gotten in 7 hours had you been breathing properly. Maybe your snoring and/or sleep apnea caused you to come out of deep, restorative sleep repeatedly all night. Maybe acid reflux prevented you from ever reaching the deepest levels of sleep. How would you know? The answer is, most likely, you wouldn't. And you wouldn't know that you didn't know unless you scrutinized your sleep in ways which I am going to teach you. The first thing to understand and accept though is that unless you have a decent amount of data about your sleep, collected with good tools, you really know very little about how you sleep.

We all sleep every night (usually) and if there is no marker or metric to tell us what a truly good night's sleep is, then what constitutes a good night's sleep, especially as time goes by, is subject to become considerably distorted. For me, it reached a point where if I were just able to sleep through the night, I thought I'd had a good night's sleep. I was wrong, and if I hadn't figured that out and done something about it, the quality of my life would have continued to deteriorate until it culminated in an early death. That is a fact.

I had already become seriously depressed, sick, and was a walking zombie. I NEVER felt 100% awake and effective, and that became disturbingly normal to me over time. I took naps during the day, medications to get to sleep and then other medications to stay awake during the day. Consistency in work, my personal life, and life in general just faded to the point where they were only a distant memory. I was an absolute mess. But, most insidiously, it all happened so *gradually* that I couldn't see the pattern that is now so obvious to me: sleep, I came to learn, was the common thread to all of these issues.

When pop singer Michael Jackson died years ago, most people couldn't understand how it had happened. When I learned many of the facts, which included his having utilized a physician administering powerful, surgical grade intravenous sedation (an overdose of which ultimately killed him) to get him to sleep, I knew immediately the position he'd gotten himself into and how it had ultimately cost him his life. A close friend of his at the time recounted Jackson saying, "If I could just get a good night's sleep...everything would be ok" That is a smoking gun. When I heard that, I knew the hole he had fallen inextricably into. I knew because I'd barely pulled myself out of it. Had I had access to the kinds of medications and people Michael Jackson had, I'd likely be dead as well.

There is a point where sleep deprivation and/or poor sleep quality can spiral dangerously out of control. In my case, I'd gone from an occasional dose of a leading prescription sleep medication to 3x that dosage and then even more, with diminishing results. On top of that, I took powerful wakefulness meds during the day and occasionally anti-anxiety meds to calm myself down. One day, I suddenly took inventory of all the things I was ingesting to get to sleep and stay awake. Recognizing what I was doing left me thinking of people like actor Heath Ledger, who had recently died from an overdose of prescription meds. In that moment, one of the most pivotal insights flashed through my mind and I felt a cold shiver of dread as I thought: *"This is how people inadvertently kill themselves – unintentional interactions from multiple drugs in their system."* I knew it was time to find a different way to get where I needed to go, and I stopped taking the medications I was using immediately. Make no mistake about it, sleep medications are deadly and should be avoided. 4 years ago, my ex-girlfriend was found dead alone in her home after an overdose of Ambien. She too had fallen into the spiral that took Michael Jackson and countless others.

The erosion of what we've come to believe is a good night's sleep is a glacially slow process. Most of us sleep just fine from birth until we are into our teens when unnecessarily early school start times begin to destroy our sleep pattern at a critical developmental age – something that is only now beginning to be recognized and corrected around the country and world for the first time. For the majority of us, the toll taken from not sleeping well doesn't really start to show up until our 30's or so. Think about it: when you were a child or a teenager, do you ever remember having an issue with sleep or even thinking about it, much less on a regular basis? (other than when being dragged from bed sometime before 7AM to get to school on time or before 11 AM during summer vacation...) For most of us, it was just like a light switch got switched off and nothing registered until we awoke up the next morning and picked up right where we left off; a wondrous, restorative intermission between energy filled days. That distant memory is what sleep is *supposed* to be like, even now.

The only sleep issue I ever recall as a youth was the occasional argument with my parents about wanting to stay up later or being too excited to fall asleep at the normal time on Christmas Eve and then waking up at 4 AM on Christmas morning to sneak down and see what had been left under the tree for me. Other than that, I remember nothing about the sleep of my youth. Nothing except, that is, having a lot more dreams – longer, more vivid, detailed dreams; the kind of dreams one should be having when they are experiencing the type of sleep cycle that allows for natural restorative processes to revitalize their brain and body. I'll wager you remember something similar.

It was during high school that I first remember myself or others falling asleep in class, sleeping extra on weekends to make up for lost hours during the week, or experiencing any significant fatigue. College was more of the same and to a much greater degree, particularly when coupled with frequent late nights out.

So now, think about those nights of sleep as a child, when you went to bed at a set time and recall nothing but incredibly realistic dreams until you woke up the next morning instantly ready to go. Compare that to last night, and I will ask you again: How did you sleep last night?

The fact of the matter is that I would have just gone on thinking I slept fine night after night, like many people do, if something hadn't happened that woke me up (sorry...) to the clear and definite fact that although I *thought* I was sleeping fine, I was *not.* It was this realization that took me on a 15+ year journey to find out why I couldn't get a good night's sleep. It took me a lot of work, research, testing, and experimentation to learn what has gotten me to where I can now sleep nearly perfectly every night. And I'm going to share my secrets with you, so that you can do the same in just a matter of days or weeks. I hope you are ready for a dramatic improvement in the quality of your life because, after you know what I know, you will never sleep the same again.

The War On Sleep

"Sleep, those little slices of death – how I loathe them."

-Edgar Allan Poe

The sentiments of American author Edgar Allan Poe on sleep, as expressed above in the mid-1800s, are not uncommon among many Americans even today. One might well argue that the attitude he expressed was well ahead of its time. It may also very well be one of the factors that contributed to Mr. Poe's poor health and early death at the young age of 40 in 1849.

There is no doubt about it: Americans are engaged in a battle against proper rest. It is a foolish, losing battle that is taking a massive toll on us both individually and as a society. We are losing fast. The signs are everywhere.

Human beings today, on average, get about 120 minutes less sleep per night than we did just 50 years ago.[1] Bear in mind that is on average – which means that a significant portion of us are getting even less – 2 or 3 hours less is not uncommon. It is almost a certainty that we are the only species on Earth for which this is occurring, except for those which we also disrupt with our sleep cheating activities. (ALL known species on earth sleep.) In the past 150 years, numerous things which were previously uncommon have now become epidemics: heart disease, diabetes, depression, mental illness, stroke, cancers, Alzheimer's Disease and obesity. These are, in fact, what most of us are destined to die from. Why? And why are we sleeping less? Is there a connection?

The answer lies in what I call The War On Sleep, which we began waging over 100 years ago and have pushed to the breaking point today. It is a losing battle in which we have suffered major casualties and gained nothing but decreased quality of life and earlier death. We have incurred huge losses both as a society and as individuals which we may only be just starting to comprehend, and the time to surrender and make peace is well at hand. For too long now, we have been of the opinion that sleep is unnecessary, a needles luxury to be cut wherever other things take priority. We wanted to get more done, but never knew what the cost was until it became extremely high – just how high, we are still tabulating.

How and why we began this mindless assault on proper sleep, no one can really say, but by looking at the factors which contributed to it we can get an idea that it roughly coincides with the industrialization of our society. The major factors which began the war around 150 years ago (roughly 2 lifetimes in today's metrics) are:

1) The availability of electric lighting. Our ancestors, even with fire, had a rigid cycle of darkness during which it was extremely difficult to do any productive things. So, at night, they slept like they were intended to, when they were intended to. Caves and huts are dark at night, as is the savannah. Fire, even used all night for warmth, gives off a low red spectrum form of light. Anyone who has slept by a camp fire or fireplace knows it is actually soothing, dim, and hard to read or do detailed work by this type of light, in contrast to the blinding spectra of artificial light (mostly white /blue in frequency) that we use in our homes today. A fire, unlike an electric light, is warm, soothing, and comfortable to sleep by – it is actually conducive to sleep for most people. Research has concluded that you will fall asleep by a fire more easily than not.[2] What's more, fires kept nocturnal predators and

---

[1] National Geographic Naked Science: Dead Tired

[2] Dana Lynn Christopher, "Hearth and campfire influences on arterial blood pressure: defraying the costs of the social brain through fireside relaxation."

insects like mosquitos away, allowing our ancestors to sleep securely as well as comfortably. We continued this tradition using fireplaces and lanterns and other such sources of contained flames well into the 1800s and, for the most part, kept normal circadian sleep cycles like most other animals on Earth. Until we didn't.

2)   Shift work. Since the beginning of the industrial revolution, we have been pushing back the frontiers of darkness to be productive closer to 24 waking hours than 12 and, consequently, have reduced our average sleep cycle. Shift work, first made possible at that time and now commonplace amongst a large portion of society, greatly increased this phenomenon. With industrial factories to run and electric lighting so we could see, there was no longer any barrier to working 24 hours a day, and Pandora's box was thus opened. We have been paying the price for this ever since.

3)   Modern communications and devices. We are now never truly in a state of being alone and minimally subject to disturbance as our ancestors were during their sleeping hours. Our sleep time is in danger of interruption at any second by cell phones, sirens, loud vehicles, neighbors, aircraft flying over, email, texts and on and on. If one does not actively protect one's sleep time against such looming intrusions, all it takes is a single disruption of REM sleep to induce days of damage to sleep quality. Maybe even weeks. The ability to sleep in a calm, quiet environment has become, for many, the exception as opposed to the rule.

4)   Lack of respect for sleep. Every known species on Earth sleeps. Sleep is clearly NOT an unnecessary process or it would have been evolved out long ago. Clearly, species with perfect evolutionary records, such as humans, require sleep to achieve this position. Animals respect sleep – just watch them. Given the opportunity, their natural inclination is to sleep when it's time to do so, not stay up and watch tv, play, or work. Via an innate mechanism, they respect sleep and keep it's time cycle regular like clockwork.

Evolutionary Psychology Nov 11, 2014

Even when surrounded by humans and their unnatural influences and patterns. Who hasn't stayed up working late and glanced over at their dog who was sleeping away soundly since his usual bedtime? Most humans do not respect sleep in this way, quite the opposite in fact. We have deluded ourselves into thinking that sleep is unnecessary, that sleeping is akin to weakness, and that, to succeed, sleep must be defeated in exchange for ever longer hours and more work. "There's plenty of time to sleep when you're dead," is a well-worn cliché we have all heard. A more accurate rendition might be, "There' s plenty of time to die when you don't sleep." Because lack of sleep is, indeed, a means to an earlier death as an end – much more so than we ever believed up until now.

Sleep deprivation very quickly takes a toll on cognitive functions and attention. In as little as 16 hours without sleep, a typical day for many, a person's performance level degrades and very closely resembles that of someone with a blood alcohol content of .08 percent – legally drunk in most places. Would you drive in that condition? By 24 hours, it nearly doubles to .15% equivalency. And yet, how many people are doing things that endanger their and others' lives in this condition every day? We know not to do this with alcohol, so why don't we know not to do it with sleep? Our thinking needs to change.

It is estimated that fatigue is responsible for 20% of all workplace accidents. Shockingly, in the health care industry, a survey of medical interns by Harvard Medical School found that 1 in 5 interns admitted to making a fatigue related error which resulted in the injury of a patient and 1 in 20 interns reported *making a fatigue related error that resulted in the death of a patient.*[3] This is nothing short of shocking, particularly *in the medical field where an understanding of the importance of sleep should be a given.* It is not and, rather than teaching medical students to respect the need for sleep and never treat a patient when they are not properly rested, our medical institutions instead feed interns the mistaken belief that the answer is to attempt to train them to think under sleep deprived conditions. We don't let bus drivers drive or pilots fly sleep deprived, so why in the *hell* do we allow doctors to treat critically ill patients while in such condition? That intern or resident who treats you in the ER next time you go there may very possibly be working under the equivalent of a .15 or greater blood alcohol level – legally drunk. Sound like something you'd want to do? I sure wouldn't. It is in truth little more than a form of hazing or forcing new MDs to 'pay dues' based on tradition and it needs to end immediately. It is killing people needlessly; there are numerous incidents on record where sleep deprived medical personnel driving home from 24 hour+ work shifts have killed innocent drivers when they lost control of their vehicles and caused fatal accidents after falling asleep at the wheel.

---

[3] National Geographic Naked Science: Dead Tired

Sleep deprivation ("drowsy driving") in the US is responsible for *1 in every 4* motor vehicle accidents. But that's nothing: in the US, an astonishing *250,000 people fall asleep at the wheel of a motor vehicle every day.*[4] More than 1500 die as a result each year. The statistics are likely far worse, but being tired isn't something we can test for like drugs or alcohol. In June of 2014, comedian Jimmy Mack was killed and actor Tracy Morgan of the television show '30 Rock' was critically injured when their vehicle was struck by an 18-wheel Walmart truck whose (professional) driver had not slept in over 24 hours. Every day, similar accidents happen taking the lives of less famous people, we just don't hear about them as they aren't as "newsworthy".

The American Academy of Sleep Medicine and the US Centers for Disease Control (CDC) both consider sleep deprivation to be, and I quote, "A disease which has reached epidemic proportions." The CDC has called this chronic sleep loss a *public health epidemic*. Let that sink in for a minute. The fact is that this sleep deprivation epidemic will kill orders of magnitude more people than COVID-19, but it will happen much more slowly so it is not obvious. It is, however, the FAR worse health crisis. It will kill most people reading these words. If you find that disturbing, you absolutely should, and you are in good company. As we will learn in the pages ahead, the top 3 killers of both men and women in the US are directly relatable to sleep disorders which may indicate, and I believe it does, that sleep deprivation may in fact be, as a root causation, *the number one killer of men and women in the US.* I'll say that again succinctly for emphasis: ***Sleep deprivation may very possibly be the number one killer of men and women in the US.***

My Long, Difficult Relationship with Sleep

---

[4] National Geographic Naked Science: Dead Tired

If you are reading this book knowing that you have some kind of a problem with your sleep, congratulations: you are a step ahead of most people with sleep issues. The vast majority who have one are not even aware of it, much less trying to correct it. I was one of those people until about 15 years ago.

The reason for this is very easy to understand once you know it, but extremely elusive before that point. Like any number of progressive dysfunctions, sleep issues are not something that hit you overnight with full, obvious force; they are a *very* gradual, slowly accumulating and evolving phenomena that build up at a snail's pace over a very, very long time and may manifest symptoms in numerous ways. If you've ever had an injury or condition that got very gradually worse over a very long time and then was suddenly alleviated by some medication or surgery or other intervention, you may have been astounded at how bad it had gotten and that you only realized how debilitating it had been after it was alleviated. This is not uncommon – humans are VERY adaptable to even very painful conditions that evolve slowly over a long period of time. This is one of the inherent characteristics that has allowed all of us who are alive today on planet Earth to survive and evolve. Those who lacked this capacity are long gone. We adapt or we perish.

Sleep issues are perhaps the most insidious of these types of progressive maladies. They tend to come on in our late twenties and build up at a glacial pace until, by the time we are in our 50s and beyond, they have destroyed the quality of our lives or killed us. Age, in and of itself, is not something that should necessarily have any negative effect on quality of sleep, yet look how many people over age 30 look and feel tired much of the time as compared to those under 30. Kids rarely snore, older people do all the time.

I've never seen anyone under 30 with a CPAP (Continuous Positive Airway Pressure – more on that later) mask on. That which we have grown to believe is an effect is, in fact, much more of a cause than we had any idea. That is to say, aging doesn't necessarily lead to bad sleep, but bad sleep unquestionably accelerates aging. Sleep disorders extract a cumulative toll on an extremely gradual basis and, if undetected and left to continue, shorten our lives while destroying their quality. This is fact, not theory. I'll say it once more to be perfectly clear: poor sleep shortens your life and destroys its quality right up until the end of your foreshortened life. We all know someone who looks 10 or more years younger than most people their age and someone who looks 10 or more years older than most their age. Ever wonder why?

I didn't know there was anything wrong with my sleep 15 years ago. I had however come to realize that sleep was crucial to me because if, for example, I stayed up much too long at a stretch or was negatively affected by jet lag, I suffered severely. I came to respect sleep, but I thought it was just an aspect of aging or my own personal physiology. In my 20s, I could work a 10 hour day on a Friday, spend 2 hours driving 45 miles from my home in Orange County to Los Angeles to stay out partying with friends until 1 or 2 in the morning, drive home arriving back at 3 or 4 AM, and then do it again Saturday night without any issue returning to a normal work week on Monday. Somewhere along the line in my late 30s, that ability disappeared. I thought everyone needed and would be better off with a nap or two during the day like me. I thought plenty of people snored and drooled while sleeping and that those were merely indications of sound sleep. I had no clue that my sleep quality was terrible and only getting worse and that, in time, I was headed for a terrible quality of life followed by an early death, despite taking the best possible care of my health I knew how to. The "eureka moment" came for me sometime in 2005. Like many such revelatory moments, it has an interesting story behind it.

I Meet A Model at A Party

It was sometime in the fall of 2005. I was at one of those house parties in the Hollywood Hills area of Los Angeles where a lot of (mostly entertainment industry) people who don't know each other meet in a beautiful house on a lovely night and enjoy the evening with open bars on a deck overlooking the city lights. I found myself waiting in a short line in a hallway for the restroom facing a stunning blonde, blue eyed girl from Germany.

We talked for a few minutes and ended up getting together sometime a few days later. A date ended at my house and we were getting along well, if you take my meaning, when she produced some cocaine from her purse and offered me some. Now, I have had pretty much zero interest in recreational drugs since about age 24 but, living in Los Angeles, this is something that comes up from time to time if you partake in night life at any level. Any other time, that would probably have been the end of the conversation. But, I'd had a couple of drinks, was having a good time, and this girl was 10 years younger than me and looked like a supermodel, so I didn't feel like making waves and decided it would be one of those rare times when all variables were just right for me to say, "screw it, why not?!" So, I said sure, and off we went. A bad decision was about to have a rare very good outcome.

The main reason I didn't really want to mess with cocaine, having had experience with it in the past[5], was that I knew I was probably going to be destroying my night's sleep and, at this point in my life, I'd come to learn that a bad night of sleep would haunt me for several days until I got evened out again somehow. I once read a brilliant quote from Ronald Reagan who said, "Middle age is when, presented with two temptations, you choose the one that will get you home and to bed by 10 PM." Ain't THAT the truth. But the trade-off this time was a night with a supermodel, so it was an easy decision. I did my best to ingest as little of the drug as possible – probably just one small dose in each nostril and that was it. Having not touched it in a decade and, as such, having no tolerance for it whatsoever, that was plenty.

I went to sleep somewhere around 2 AM. I dropped into bed expecting to stare at the ceiling listening to my heart race as I'd done too many times in college. But that didn't happen. Instead, I somehow drifted off to sleep quickly and I woke up the next morning around 10 AM feeling more rested and awake than I had in at least a decade. *How was that possible?* Cocaine had always been a ticket to a lousy night unable to sleep until the sun was coming up, followed by a day of feeling terrible, in my experience. Something had happened that had given me my best night of sleep in many years, and I had to find out what and why. This was not a small deal – it was tangibly significant – I felt *amazing*. Something major had happened here. I'd had a magical night of restorative sleep that made me feel like a million dollars. Why? How? It was immediately obvious that I'd been sleeping very, very poorly without knowing it and that a much, much better night of sleep was possible. I HAD to know how.

---

[5] In college, I briefly had a roommate who was a cocaine dealer. He was an NCAA level wrestler in great physical condition. A few years back, I Googled him only to find out he'd died of a heart attack at age 37. Beware: cocaine is a terrible drug which does lasting damage that may not come back to haunt you for decades. Stay away from it. Another friend of mine, a woman in perfect health, recently died at age 40 of an aortic dissection after using cocaine.

And thus began my 15 year quest for better sleep.

Section 2: The Problem

"If I could just get a good night's sleep, everything would be ok."

-Michael Jackson

Why Do We Sleep?

Until quite recently, the answer(s) to this seemingly simple question had mostly eluded medical science. The short answer is, because we have to. Every known species on Earth sleeps. Why would every land animal on Earth evolve to need to spend 1/3 or more of its hours every day in a state which, out on the savannah, makes it an easy target to become another animal's dinner while contributing seemingly nothing to hunting, gathering, nor finding a mate? The answer is it wouldn't unless there was a VERY good reason.

If you go to most any good survival training course, one of the first things you will learn are these three critical resources and how to manage them – air, water, and food. These are the 3 elements necessary to sustain human life, right? Or are they….?

A good survival school will teach you very early on that you can survive approximately:
3 minutes without air
3 days without water
3 weeks without food

We say approximately because the exact number depends on many variables, such as your body mass index, height and weight, level of initial hydration, etc. Regardless, the numbers are pretty similar for everyone any way you slice it.

However, there is another resource which you CANNOT live without that is never in this list – not that I have ever seen at least – and that is sleep. It's position in this list is probably going to surprise you. The absolute fact is that you can go NO MORE THAN 10 DAYS without sleep. That's right, sleep is more important than food. Stories you hear from people about how they can go weeks without sleeping are just that – stories. Science has proven otherwise conclusively. So, here is what the complete resource guide really looks like:

You can survive approximately:
3 minutes without air
3 days without water
10 days without sleep
3 weeks without food

This is really not accurate, though. The fact of the matter is that no human can, on their own, go anywhere near 10 days without sleeping. Your body WILL sleep, whether you know it or not, long before then by doing what is known as 'micro-sleep'. More about that later. For practical purposes, you might as well throw another 3 into the guideline because you will pretty much never, without significant chemical or other aides, go anywhere near 3 days without sleep. But, for now, we will just keep it at 10 until science completes debunking that.

So, why is sleep so important, and why do most people not know this?

Sleep is something I never thought about. All that mattered was that I did it when I needed to. Because I only have access to my own experience, I never had any idea as to how other people felt when they were tired, how they felt when they first woke up, what time they went to bed, what time they fell asleep, etc. Like the vast majority of people, it just never occurred to me to wonder about it. Only recently has this information become easily collectible and available for study.

It wasn't until my 30s that I began to question my own sleep. I became aware, mostly through girlfriends, that I regularly snored when I slept. That didn't really register any significance to me other than to apologize. One girlfriend had experience with this issue from her ex and had earplugs she'd use whenever she slept over. Living alone most of my life with my dog, this never really created any problem, so I barely gave it a second thought.

The thing about sleep quality that makes it so hard to quantify is that it is both subjective and relative for each person. Until recently, nobody (other than maybe a subject in a sleep lab) kept daily, quantitative records on their sleep quality. If I ask a person how they slept last night, they will most likely answer based simply upon how they are feeling or how they felt when they woke up that morning. They're not, for example, likely to have some quantified idea of how they slept last night, compare that night's sleep against all other nights they can remember and answer according to how that night's sleep stood up against all others. We generally tend to slog through life not having any idea of how our sleep quality is until or unless it becomes so bad as to be intolerable. Even then, most of us then resort to methods to quickly assess it which are generally inaccurate. If our sleep quality diminishes very gradually over time, as it does for many of us, we become accustomed to a terrible night's sleep feeling "normal" and would never really know the difference unless by some stroke of luck we had a terrible night's sleep (maybe our norm) one night followed by a fantastic night the next. This might make one say, "Hey, wow, that was a WAY better night of sleep than I've had in ages? How did that happen?" Unfortunately, few of us are lucky enough to find ourselves in such a situation as I did.

It is only recently that the answer to the question of why we sleep has come to light. Perhaps the most significant finding to date is that, during sleep, the body circulates cerebrospinal fluid through the brain some 20 times faster than during awake hours. This circulation has been discovered to serve the purpose of carrying waste products out of the brain for disposal – waste products that are produced during normal cognitive activity and creation of neural pathways. Without this "cleanup" cycle, your ability to perform cognitively during your next waking period is significantly negatively impacted. Quite literally, your brain needs sleep to perform, and good sleep to perform at a high level.

In all other parts of the body, the waste products produced by normal processes are collected and removed by the lymphatic system. It was long a mystery how the brain, isolated from the lymphatic system by the blood-brain barrier, was able to flush out any accumulated wastes. Now we know that that the CS fluid hyper-circulation during sleep accomplishes this – it is an engineering marvel of nature.

The primary waste matters that are flushed during this process are proteins known as Amyloid Beta and Tau. These proteins in the brain coalesce into plaques on neural structures which have been shown to interfere with cognitive function, not unlike how rust on wires impairs electrical signals. These plaques have been linked conclusively to a number of diseases, most notably Alzheimer's disease, Chronic Traumatic Encephalopathy (CTE) and diabetes. Over the past 10 years, significant links have been found between diabetes and Alzheimer's Disease. While these links and what is cause versus effect are not fully understood as yet, the links are undeniable. What we know for certain is that the factors which lead to diabetes also lead to and contribute to plaque formation in the brain and associated dementias, most notably Alzheimer's Disease. Taking measures that limit risk of diabetes at this point is recognized as being preventative of AD as well and getting proper sleep is now recognized to be a major one of those measures.

In a nutshell, Tau and Amyloid Beta plaques accumulating in the brain and impairing cognitive function are now conclusively known to be caused by both head trauma (chronicled in the excellent film "Concussion") and sleep deprivation. Yes, depriving yourself of proper sleep has the same effect on your brain as being repeatedly hit in the head hard enough to cause a concussion. My stepfather died a few years back in his late 80s. He played football at Notre Dame in the 1940s – the days of leather helmets – and worked long days sleeping short hours most of his life. He died of Alzheimer's disease after a 5+ year deterioration.

This is not really a surprise when you think about it in the proper context. There is no doubt that the brain is an extremely high-performance machine. High-performance machines, such as Formula One racing engines, are NOT designed to have long service cycles. They are, necessarily, built for periods of high performance alternated with regular maintenance cycles to maintain peak performance. Shorten, degrade, or skip the maintenance cycle even once and the wear and tear quickly begin to take a toll on the system, affecting performance and longevity. If this continues unabated, the system's performance degrades and it ultimately fails. If you run that formula one engine beyond its intended cycle without downtime and maintenance, it will fail. Even a lower performance, more ruggedized car will fail, given enough neglect. Compare this to your brain, which is the highest performing unit in any known animal, and it becomes clear that the brain is not designed to sustain lots of neglect. That oil circulating through a Formula One Engine is much like the fluid in your brain. It keeps the parts moving smoothly and gathers up waste bits of metal and dirt, all of which need to be flushed out before the next operational cycle. Skip that maintenance cycle, and next operation cycle will be lower performing. Don't stop for the maintenance cycle and you are on a countdown to engine failure – catastrophic engine failure. Conversely, perform regular proper maintenance, and performance can be kept near optimal for an extremely long time. The analogy is, in reality, very similar.

An amazing fact is that our brains, which constitute only at best 2% of our body mass, use fully 20% of the calories we consume for operation. That is nothing short of amazing and illustrates how much work our brains do. In short, sleep is how your brain flushes its waste products out, making it one of the most, if not the most, critical biological functions there is. There are organs you can survive and even thrive without, but the brain is **not** one of them. Hence, sleep is not something to be shortchanged – it serves a critical function.

How We Die Now

As striking as that evidence is, it is far from all we have learned recently. In a study with staggering implications, research published in the January 2014 journal Cancer Research found the following:

Poor-quality sleep, marked by frequent awakenings, can speed cancer growth, increase tumor aggressiveness and dampen the immune system's ability to control or eradicate early cancers.[6]

Are you paying attention yet? Because there's more. In 2012, researchers at the University of Alabama, Birmingham discovered that adults who routinely sleep less than 6 hours per night are *four times* more likely to suffer a stroke.

A number of studies have also been done researching links between heart disease and sleep. It will now probably not surprise you to learn that strong evidence has also been found linking these as well. One such study presented as part of a World Health Organization program followed men for 14 years beginning in 1994 and found that two thirds (63%) of subjects who had a heart attack also had sleep disorders. Overall, the risk of heart disease was calculated to be 2 to 2.6 x greater in the subjects with sleep issues. The study also found that stroke risk was 1.5 to 4 times higher, conforming to the previously mentioned research.

---

[6] John Easton "Fragmented Sleep Accelerates Cancer Growth" U Chicago News January 27, 2014

Let's just stop right here for a minute and consider what we just read. In the last few years, research has **conclusively** linked sleep disorders with Alzheimer's disease, diabetes, stroke, heart disease, and cancer. That is a *staggering* discovery. And it explains why we are now dying primarily of these things instead of old age and other more naturally explicable causes. It may not have been obvious in the past, but today it is: sleep deprivation is what we are now mostly dying from. We waged a War On Sleep, and we lost. Badly. We just haven't realized we were beaten and surrendered yet. Contrary to a popularly parroted cliché, sitting is NOT the new smoking; **poor sleep** is the new smoking.

Take a look at the top 10 causes of death 120 years ago versus today:

Leading Causes of Death in the United States (CDC)

1900	2020
1) Pneumonia	1) Heart Disease
2) Tuberculosis	2) Cancers
3) Diarrhea, enteritis, intestinal ulceration	3) Accidents
4) Heart Disease	4) Chronic respiratory diseases
5) Intracranial lesions	5) Stroke
6) Nephritis (kidney failure/disease)	6) Alzheimer's Disease
7) Accidents	7) Diabetes
8) Cancers / tumors	8) Influenza / pneumonia
9) Senility	9) Nephritis/ nephrotic syndrome
10) Diphtheria	10) Suicide (mental illness / depression)

Strikingly, with the exception of influenza which still kills some 60,000 Americans each year, infectious diseases have been wiped from the list entirely. Diabetes, which was not on the 1900 list at all, is now number 7. With the exception of influenza, sleep can be linked or strongly linked to all of the other 9 current leading causes of death, including accidents and likely the inflammation involved in nephritis. In some instances, as will be discussed ahead, these causes may be intertwined by sleep in the same individual multimodally. It is also highly likely that sleep contributes to influenza deaths via diminished immune response in sleep deprived persons, so really it is likely related to all the leading causes of death. It is my belief that today's leading causes of death are all tied to poor sleep in most individuals.

Circadian Cycle

Circadian cycle is an innate awareness in living things of the time of day and certain biological functions that are scheduled to automatically occur at different times throughout the day, every day, for our entire lives. Not only is circadian cycle programmed into every living thing on Earth, it is actually programmed into every cell of every living thing. We are only just beginning to understand it's incredible and all-encompassing importance.

It is not an accident that animals on Earth, wherever humans have not interfered with their lives, do not suffer from sleep disorders while humans do. Animals living on Earth today are living their lives pretty much the same way they were thousands and even millions of years ago. Specifically, they are governed by their surroundings and nature above all else. Even our domesticated pets like dogs and cats adhere to these drives; they eat when they are hungry (to the extent that they are able to), sleep when they are tired, work or hunt during certain times, and sleep at night. (Note: cats are nocturnal hunters and naturally sleep more during the day and are active at night. Dogs are mostly the opposite.) It is interesting to note that a degree of intermittent fasting occurs naturally in this cycle as the availability of food in the wild is highly variable. This has become a much-studied area of evolutionary biochemistry in recent years. Despite the fact that our pets are exposed to the same unnatural stimuli that we are (lights, sounds, communications, etc.) they "switch off" the world when it is time to sleep and, in doing so, adhere to their natural rhythms far better in general than we do. Because we humans no longer do this, we suffer the consequences. Every cell in the human body is aware of the circadian cycle, and research has shown conclusively that the disruption of this cycle leads to health problems. The following excellent illustration shows what a normal 24-hour human circadian rhythm pattern looks like when humans live the way nature intended:

Human 24-hour Circadian Rhythm[7]

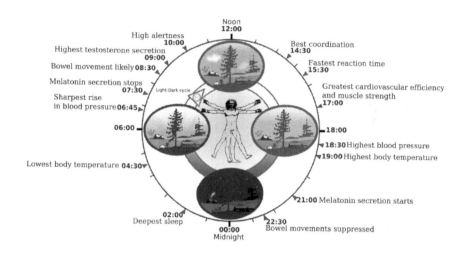

[7] Image used under terms granted via GNU Free Documentation License under the Creative Commons Attribution-Share Alike license(s). Details available at https://commons.wikimedia.org/wiki/File:Biological_clock_human.svg

Some of these things may be familiar to you already, such as having high testosterone levels in the morning or low body temperature around 4 AM. However, many of these things are unknown to many of us, such as melatonin secretion starting at 9PM and dropping off around 8AM. One major reason for this is that the secretion of melatonin in humans is regulated in large part by the amount of light reaching the retinas in our eyes. If we are still exposed to light long after dark, melatonin secretion may be inhibited or not start at all. This is but one of the many ways we inadvertently disrupt our normal sleep patterns. As such, the regulation of exposure to certain types of light after normal sunset time until sunrise can be utilized in restoring normal circadian cycle. This is something that I utilize quite a bit.

The Stages of Sleep

While it might seem that sleep is a simple, binary affair where a person is either asleep or awake at any given time, nothing could be further from the truth. There are several different stages of sleep characterized by different levels of activity in the brain and different depths of sleep. It is not really necessary for us to get into detail about these different stages, but what is important to know is that when you are sleeping properly you will cycle through the different stages of sleep about once every 90 minutes or so. If this is happening when you analyze your own sleep, then you are sleeping well and if it does not then there is an issue to address. It is also very useful to know that awakening at the top (or shallowest) level of sleep in such a cycle is significantly easier and better for us than being awakened at the middle or bottom of a cycle, both of which can be quite damaging. Good sleep metrics tools generally have the option to help you awaken within certain windows of time when you are at the top of such a cycle.

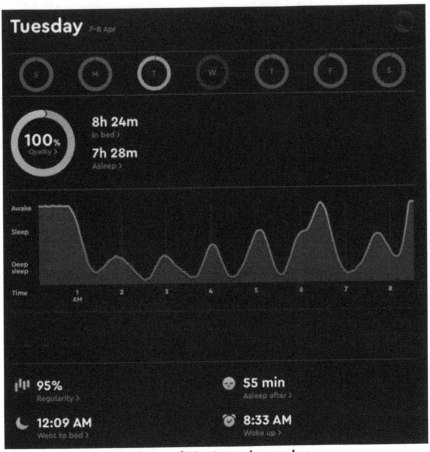

A good night of sleep with normal 90-minute sleep cycles.

The Dangers of Sleep Deprivation

Over the past several decades, sleep has become a major topic of scientific inquiry. At the University of Pennsylvania School of Medicine's Sleep Lab alone, over 10,000 full 24 hour awake/asleep cycles have been simulated in patients living for extended periods in the laboratory to collect data. This single lab's tests exceed all the sleep studies ever previously conducted combined. The more research that is completed, the more conclusive links are discovered between sleep deprivation and serious health issues some of which, if untreated, end in death. There is excellent cause to believe that the epidemics of obesity, heart disease, and depression we are experiencing in the United States as of the past 5 decades or more are a direct consequence of our war on sleep.

The consequences of sleep deprivation are swift and severe. In recent years, sleep research has discovered conclusive links between sleep loss and virtually all of the leading causes of death in the United States. There can be some variation as to cause and effect in each individual circumstance, but where there is consistent sleep disturbance, these maladies are sure to follow. Where there is depression in particular, there is sleep disturbance effectively 100% of the time.

There is a vicious cycle that is induced by sleep loss in a very short period of time and the following diagram is a simple but accurate depiction of the cycle of how sleep loss destroys health over the long term and why it is very probably the root cause of our current epidemics of obesity, diabetes, and heart disease.

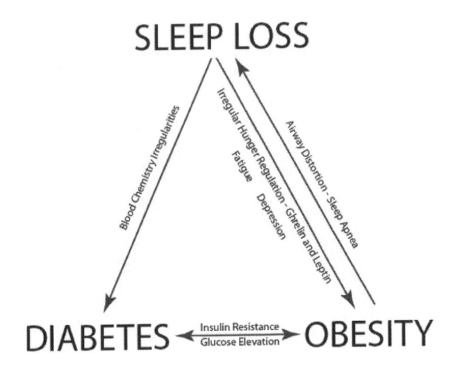

The Vicious Cycle of Sleep Loss

The cycle above works like this: After just a few nights of sleep deprivation, our bodies lose proper regulation of the hormones leptin and ghrelin, which signal us that we are hungry and full respectively. Have you ever noticed how you start getting hungry more frequently when you stay awake for long periods? This is why. Additionally, just a few nights of sleep loss can also begin moving an individual's blood chemistry into the pre-diabetic range. If the sleep loss is sustained, most people will begin to gain weight and weight gain has a pronounced effect on the airway as most people will gain weight in their neck areas fairly quickly. Overall weight gain and specific weight gain in the neck distort the airway, which is flexible and resembles the hose of a vacuum cleaner. The excess weight gains can pinch or partially collapse the airway leading to sleep apnea, snoring, and further disrupted sleep. This in turn further pushes an individual into the diabetic range promoting further weight gain. Do nothing to stop the sleep disturbance and the cycle becomes perpetual. There are many variations on these interactions and how they start, but the overall synergy and cycle is well established. To break the cycle, something has to break one side of the triangle. Often this can be done with a Continuous Positive Airway Pressure (CPAP) machine to alleviate sleep apnea/snoring until the person can recover into normal sleep and blood chemistry ranges. The rapid rate at which this interaction starts and becomes sustained is frightening – a week or less is all it takes in many otherwise perfectly healthy individuals by just cutting their sleep to 6 hours or less.

It is generally a good practice to do our best to avoid setting ourselves up with any of the sides of this deadly triangle. First and foremost, make sure you are breathing properly at night – no snoring, no sleep apnea or breathing disturbances of any kind. ***This is priority number one.*** If you are overweight, do what it takes to lose the excess weight. If you have disrupted breathing at night, get help with that and you will find that weight loss a LOT easier to achieve and sustain. If you are not allowing sufficient time for sleep – find a way to correct this. If you are diabetic or pre-diabetic, seek treatment immediately. If your work situation dictates that you cannot get a proper night's sleep, weigh whether it is worth your life to keep that job. Do whatever you need to in order to get out of this triangle of death.

Diabetes

As already mentioned, there are long known and direct connections between diabetes and sleep. In recent years, however, these links have been found to be stronger than was ever conceived before. The accumulation of cognition impairing plaques in the brain which cause Alzheimer's Disease is now strongly believed in scientific circles to be a form of type 3 diabetes – a staggering discovery. However this all pans out, sleep is known to cause amyloid and tau plaque accumulation in the brain and those protein accumulations are known to cause Alzheimer's. The links are firmly established: don't sleep and you will greatly increase your chances of Alzheimer's disease. Chronic sleep loss has also been determined to increase the risk of diabetes by up to 50%. [8]

---

[8] National Geographic Naked Science: Dead Tired

Heart Disease

While the exact mechanism between sleep loss and heart disease is still being researched, we do have a lot of the evidence as to how it works. One of the key elements is believed to be the impact of sleep loss on blood pressure. Elevated blood pressure is a known major cause of heart disease and sleep loss has been conclusively linked to elevated blood pressure.

The link between sleep deprivation and heart disease has also been quantified without knowing the exact causal mechanism. For example, a 10-year study performed by Harvard University tracked the sleep habits and health of more than 70,000 women between the ages of 45 and 65 that had no previous history of heart disease. (the leading cause of death in US women and men) In the end, 934 of these women suffered from coronary heart disease and 271 died from it. The researchers accounted for factors like age, weight and whether they smoked, then looked at the subjects' sleep patterns. Five percent of the women slept less than five hours per night. Those women were nearly *40 percent more likely* to suffer from heart disease than women who slept an average of eight hours. Women who slept more than nine hours per night were 37 percent more likely to have heart trouble. Since heart disease is the number one cause of death in America killing 23.5% of women and 25.1% of men, we would all be wise to pay close attention to the link between sleep and heart disease since it may very well be the case that lack of proper sleep is, in fact, the leading cause of death in America.

Stroke

Stroke is defined as an interruption of blood flow to the brain. Just as an interruption of blood flow to the heart is known as a heart attack, a stroke is also known as a "brain attack". In the same manner that interrupted blood flow to the heart often causes lasting tissue damage to the heart with lifelong effects, a stroke often does similar damage to the brain. Because the brain is such a large and complex organ with numerous blood supplies, the possible ways in which a stroke may damage brain function are incredibly varied as is their range of severity and permanence.

In the past 5 years, multiple university studies in both the US and Europe have found conclusive links between sleep disorders and elevated incidence of death from heart disease and stroke. In one such study published in the European Heart Journal, Professor Francesco Cappuccio from the University of Warwick Medical School explained, "If you sleep less than six hours per night and have disturbed sleep, you stand a 48 percent greater chance of developing or dying from heart disease and a 15 per cent greater chance of developing or dying of a stroke." These are sobering statistics that the vast majority of people have no awareness of.

With stroke checking in as the number 3 killer of women and the number 5 killer of men in the US, it is clear that something is likely behind the frequency of this cause of death, and sleep disturbance is, in my opinion, a leading contender.

Depression

I have never known a single person suffering from depression who was not also having sleep issues. Depression has been conclusively linked to sleep disorders in numerous studies. An inability to sleep is one of the key diagnostic indications of clinical depression. Another sign is sleeping too much.

While it is not as yet determined that an inability to sleep is a root cause of depression, it has been conclusively shown to be a contributing factor. The restorative nature of sleep to cognitive functions is a key element in healthy mental function. When one does not get proper sleep, fatigue becomes an issue, motivation decreases, and circadian rhythms become interrupted. Eating and exercise become irregular as well leading to a rather vicious cycle. We should think of sleep, eating, and exercise as the three pillars of life, because they surely are. A disruption in any one of these will have a marked impact on your quality of life. Disturbance of any two will certainly cause significant problems and make you a strong candidate for clinical depression and/or other health issues. A problem with all three will shorten and ultimately end your life while rapidly diminishing its quality. We would all do well to keep these three critical areas of life in sharp focus at all times and, when any one falls into an unacceptable state, give it immediate corrective attention.

I personally keep track of my state in these three areas on a daily basis by assigning them a score from 1 to 10, with 10 being best. On a white board in my office, I have the column headings D S and E for Diet, Sleep, and Exercise. Each morning, I update the number under each like this:

S	D	E
6	7	7

If any number gets to 6 or less, I take *immediate* action to raise it. This could be dropping everything to go to the gym after missing it for 4 days, or going to the grocery store to get all the food I need to plan the week's meals, or just to stop and eat something. If sleep is the issue, I look at what time I've been getting to bed, what my sleep metrics look like, and what I can change to get back on track. It's very simple, but quantifying your 3 essential states in this manner gives you a solid foundation on which to take small corrective actions as needed well before major actions are required. That is how to improve the quality of your sleep and, moreover, your life on a long-term basis.

Unintentional Injuries / Death

Accidents leading to injury or death might seem like something that are not a great cause for concern, until one examines them statistically. In the US, accidents (of all kinds, not just motor vehicle) are the number 3 killer of men and the number 6 killer of women.

In a shocking statistic from the Division of Sleep Medicine at Harvard Medical School, a staggering 250,000 people fall asleep at the wheel while driving in the US *every day*. When one contemplates all of the potentially dangerous or deadly tasks we all engage in every day from driving to walking near traffic to working with power tools, etc., the potential for sleep deprivation to injure or kill a staggering number of us each year becomes readily apparent. Worker fatigue accounts for 1/5 of all workplace accidents. One place in which sleep deprivation has been the norm for decades for reasons I fail to comprehend, hospitals, harbor additional frightening statistics. Interns and residents in the US work up to 100 hours per week, which is absolutely egregiously irresponsible. Why, in of all places the medical community, this flagrant abuse of and lack of respect for proper sleep is tolerated and perpetuated absolutely mystifies and disgusts me. We do not allow people in similar positions who hold innocent lives in their hands, such as pilots, to do this, so why on Earth would we allow doctors to do so? In July 2014 in the wake of ever-growing evidence of sleep deprivation being involved in highway accidents involving trucks, the US DOT announced that commercial truck drivers would start being screened for sleep apnea. This is a bold step in the right direction which will save lives and raise awareness. Your doctor, your pilot, the driver of the 18-wheeler next to you, these are just a few of the people who should NEVER be working while sleep deprived, and it is high time we started making sure that ALL of them are not.

Section 3: The Solution

"There's no use talking about the problem unless you talk about the solution."

-Betty Williams

Metrics

"What gets measured gets managed"

-Peter Drucker

A wise person once said, "If you don't know where you are going, any road will take you there." You may have noticed, if you were paying careful attention, that I have told you I began my sleep research some 15 years ago and yet, if you look at my sleep graph, I have had the majority of my improvement in the last five years. Why? One very good reason: personal sleep metrics. The ability to use equipment to measure, track, and quantify your sleep quality at home every night only became available to the general public about 6 years ago. This marked a huge turning point in my personal sleep research and today I have just passed the 2000 mark of recorded nights of my own sleep data. We cannot solve a problem without clearly defining it, so you will need to collect data on your own sleep to improve your sleep. Anything else would be a half-measure, and those are something one cannot engage in and expect favorable results. You must determine where you need to go before setting out to get there.

Before sleep measuring devices and programs became available, most attempts at sleep improvement were judged subjectively. As you know from my description in the early pages of this book, however good a person's intentions may be, an individual's self-reported sleep quality is generally worthless. While I had been making some degree of progress during the first 9 years, and some of it was definitely quantifiable, without question I made the most massive strides only after personal sleep metrics became available. Those improvements continue to this very day. You have a HUGE advantage to improve your sleep compared to me when I started: you can get lab quality data about your sleep from day one.

If you are going to have any possibility of improving your sleep quality, you **must** start by having some method of quantifying what the quality of your sleep is on a nightly basis. Subjective evaluation, such as writing notes about how you felt upon waking, are not enough. In order to figure out what is going on with your sleep, you will need tools with a high degree of detail and accuracy. Fortunately, these tools are now available to everyone at a very reasonable range of cost - from free to around $250. The tools I use the most and have gotten my most valuable improvements with are free and I recommend you start with these same tools. Likely you already have the smart phone or tablet needed to use them.

When I first became aware that I had a sleep issue, it was just a stroke of luck. By virtue of my one night of unimpeded breathing, I was able to observe the strong contrast between that precious good night's sleep and all of the other terrible ones that came before it and after it. It was this stark comparison that allowed me to realize that something was wrong. Unfortunately for me, this was in 2006 and at that time tools for measuring sleep quality were not available to the public. I would spend much of the next 5 years blindly doing research to improve my sleep. Today, excellent tools are available in the form of applications and sensors tied into cell phones, tablets, watches and computers which make an amazing volume of sleep feedback information available to anyone. We are moving from a time when detailed sleep data was a once or twice in a lifetime rarity obtained at great expense and inconvenience in a sleep lab to where this information is collected every night automatically at home.

The difference this makes is immense – just take a look at the data being collected at sleepcycle.com from all over the world every night. These metrics are today rapidly being recognized for their importance – so much so that newer products from Apple, Samsung and Google are being built with these biometric functionalities built in. These tools will help you improve your sleep quality quickly and effectively, and they are available for free or very reasonable prices, especially as compared to the price of $250 - $2500 for ONE night in most medical sleep study labs or home sleep studies. In addition to allowing you to get a MUCH larger sampling of data over many, many nights, the new personal metric devices also have the distinct advantage of allowing you to monitor your sleep at home in your own bed – a critical factor in my opinion.

I have, as of this writing, collected and analyzed over 2000 nights of my own sleep data while applying various things to improve my sleep and tracking the results. The result, as you can see on the back cover of this book, is an improvement of my average nightly sleep quality score from around 50% to over 90% and rising. When I started out to improve my sleep, these metrics were not available. For you, they are available before you even begin, which is such a huge advantage that I cannot even begin to convey it to you.

Before I impart anything about how to improve your sleep, you must first collect at least three nights of sleep data (preferably a week or more), to see where you are starting from. This will give you a starting point and allow you to test different sleep improvement tactics to see which work the best for you.

A lot of the people I attempt to help with their sleep stop making effort at this crucial point. DO NOT STOP HERE! Until you collect meaningful data on your sleep, you cannot take meaningful steps to improve it. *An undefined problem cannot be solved!* The tools are readily available, simple to use, and free. If you don't make the effort, you cannot possibly be serious about improving your sleep. MAKE THE EFFORT.

Tracking your sleep is as simple as my nightly routine: When I get into bed, I take my tablet and start an app called Sleep Cycle. (www.sleepcycle.om)

Sleep Cycle

By far, this is my favorite sleep tracking application and one of the single greatest breakthrough technological advances for sleep improvement (if not the single greatest) ever made. It is available for both IOS and Android devices and it is FREE. There are also some premium services available for a fee and the prices are very reasonable. Once you have loaded it onto your phone or tablet, you will see an icon like this one:

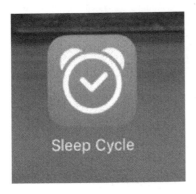

Before we get into the setup, let me explain a bit about how Sleep Cycle (and most other similar apps) work. The program runs on your device and you leave your device near your bed in a certain position all night. Your device has several sensors in it – an accelerometer, a gyroscope, light sensor, and a microphone – which are the primary sensors these programs use. Initially Sleep Cycle had users place the device on the bed to use motion sensing, but later this evolved into the device using sound sensing combined with artificial intelligence to learn your environment and then to track all activity in the room. As an engineer, I am *astonished* at how well they have developed this technology and how accurate it is. By measuring your motion and sound alone, the app can get a very good idea of what your sleep looks like. Just a note: this use of sound is done without any external or "cloud" connection, so no breach of privacy can occur. Only if you elect will samples of snoring be recorded, but these are still only stored on your device unless you elect to use cloud storage/sync. As an expert in cyber security and data privacy, I can assure you that Sleep Cycle is not something to be concerned with, particularly if you use it the way I do with device radios off.

If you add additional data from a sensor like a biometric device (Fit Bit, Apple Watch or such) you can add even more data like heart rate, body temperature, etc. and really get specific useful data. However, just your phone alone will yield a treasure trove of information. One thing – it has been shown to be disruptive to sleep to have a radio source near you when sleeping. As such, I shut off my phone or tablet's radios by putting it into airplane mode when using it to track sleep – sleep tracking programs like Sleep Cycle don't need any connection while working, which is ideal. I don't want nor need anyone contacting me while I'm sleeping anyway, and this also reduces the temptation to check messages or email if I wake up in the middle of the night – something I have trained myself to stop doing entirely over the past 6 years and which I recommend for everyone. If you MUST have your phone on at night, I suggest it be at least 10 feet away from you and you use a different device for your sleep tracker. This can be a great use for an old phone you never got rid of, or your tablet. (Note: I have no connection Sleep Cycle, but I swear by their excellent app which I have used for over 6 years now. Visit their website for some staggering statistical data they have collected from around the world over the past 10+ years.)

When I go to bed, I tell the app the approximate time I want to wake up (this is optional) – it will wait until I am in the shallowest state of sleep just before that time and play soft music to let me gently wake up – an amazing way to wake properly and I can easily continue sleeping if I wish. Then, I tell the app what factors affect my sleep for that night by checking off pre-defined 'sleep notes' which I have set up. These are things like whether or not I exercised that day, any sleep enhancing things I may have done (taking melatonin, for example) and other things which I am tracking to see if they impact my sleep positively or negatively. I then put my tablet in airplane mode to shut off the radios (which have been shown to negatively impact sleep when very close to you) and set the tablet on my bedside table. That's it. Total time, maybe 20 seconds. The app uses sound and/or motion to monitor everything going on in the room and the accuracy of the engineering is nothing short of incredible. It can filter out ambient noises like air conditioning, tv, etc. and know when you are moving, how you are breathing and what state of sleep you are in. It can also tell if you snore and record samples for you to hear while tracking total snore time. I have compared the program to a home sleep study utilizing all kinds of wired body sensors and the app was incredibly accurate and similar to the wired sleep metrics. FYI, I also put my phone in airplane mode at night – I just don't need anyone calling me at 3AM and my sleep is more important to me. Whatever happens, it can wait until after 8AM. I strongly suggest everyone get into this habit.

After 3 nights, Sleep Cycle will have enough data to sort out the sounds in your bedroom and your motions and give you very accurate sleep metrics. Now you can start working toward improving your sleep.

What A Good Night's Sleep Looks Like

In terms of sleep metrics, what does a good night's sleep look like? That's a great question. Let's take a look at one of my nightly sleep quality scores from Sleep Cycle. Every morning, I look at my sleep quality chart from the last night. Here's a really good one – my most recent 100% sleep quality score:

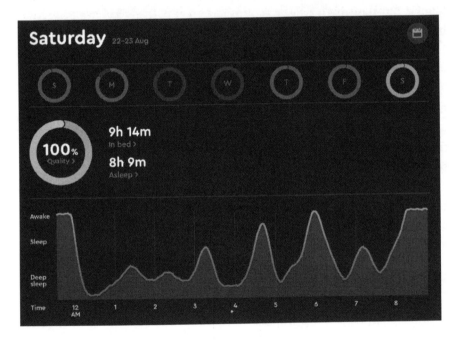

So, what makes this a good night's sleep?

First off, if we knew nothing else, the score of 100% quality tells us that this was a good night. There is variation from person to person but, for me, any sleep quality score under about 80% is not really optimal and at 70% or below I am keenly aware I have not had a good night's sleep. If, for example, I were to wake up with a 60% score, I will almost certainly feel some degree of soreness throughout my body, feel groggy, have difficulty waking, difficulty with thought process, and feel sluggish overall. I know this overall feeling right away because I long ago came to think of it as feeling like I'd been hit by a truck while I was asleep. It's a bad feeling, and it is how I will almost certainly feel with a score of 60% or less. Thankfully, I almost never have such a night anymore.

Now let's look at the graph. You will notice that I fall asleep quickly and descend into deep sleep. Then, I cycle between sleep and deep sleep about every 90 minutes for about 3-4 cycles and then steadily ascend on the upper peak of each cycle until I nearly wake up, or maybe did, around 6AM but continued sleeping for another cycle. It is quite possible that I woke up here but continued back to sleep until proper waking time – I may even have put on eyeshades to make that easier. As it appears I went to bed later than normal – around midnight - it is very likely that I put on my eyeshades and slept longer to get the proper amount of sleep. Where the chart levels off around 8AM, Sleep Cycle was set to play soft music so I would naturally wake up, and I did. While there were some challenges on this night – getting to bed late and waking up early – I was able to adjust to them and get an excellent night of sleep. This is a benefit of learning how to sleep properly and tracking progress.

This is a beautiful, classic sleep pattern and what I hope to see every night. Don't be surprised if your sleep chart for the first several nights looks NOTHING like this! For one thing, the app needs to collect some baseline data like how your movements register, how you sound, background noise to filter out, etc. for the first few nights before it can start making sense of your sleep data. Sometime around the third night or after, the chart will start to take some kind of shape. Rest assured, I do NOT always achieve a nightly chart that looks like this, and many nights I wake up once near the middle of the night (usually around 4 AM) but quickly go right back to sleep and continue until morning – no damage done. This is a common pattern and considered natural by many experts.

There are a few other things to notice on this chart: My overall sleep time was 7 hours, 53 minutes. This is fairly typical for me – I try for 7.5 to 8.5 hours which I have come to feel is optimal based on prior experience. Your number may vary a bit from mine. Also, and this is important – it is possible to get a high sleep score in less time asleep and a lower sleep quality score in more time asleep. We are measuring quality, not quantity, and time is just one factor. Generally, my best sleep quality occurs in a 7-8 hour block of sleep. Once you have collected enough data, you will know what is optimal for you.

What A Bad Night's Sleep Looks Like

Just to show you how much I have improved my sleep since I started, here is one of my earliest night's charts recorded in October of 2013 (Sleep Cycle looked a bit different back then, but the same major elements are there):

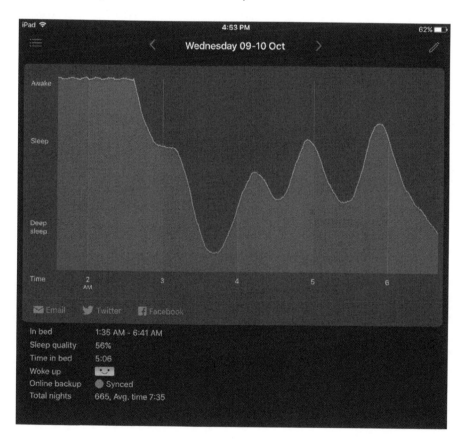

As you can see, this was a terrible night with a 56% sleep quality. While I cannot recall that specific night, I know from experience I must have felt like death the next day just by looking at that chart. Why I recorded waking up happy is surely a mistake on my part! In some countries as of this writing (Saudi Arabia comes to mind), this is an average sleep score among most of the people voluntarily submitting data with Sleep Cycle. (!) I shudder to think what a society of people sleeping like this must be like.

A Word About Sleep Studies

Before personal sleep metric trackers were available, laboratory sleep studies, generally requiring a physician's referral, were the only tool available for assessing sleep.

Sleep studies are a laboratory-controlled procedure in which a subject spends a night in a dedicated facility, usually in a hospital or outpatient facility, and has all aspects of their sleep monitored and subsequently analyzed. This can be a great tool for determining how you are sleeping (or not) and why.

Unfortunately, sleep studies, like many things, have a wide variability in their quality and many people I have encountered, including myself, had significant problems with sleep that were not picked up in sleep studies. Why?

I can only comment about my particular experience since it is the only one I was present for. The minute I saw the room where I would be sleeping, I knew there was going to be a huge problem. The office was three stories up in a medical building near a busy major street intersection in Los Angeles and the actual sleeping room was in a corner office with windows on two walls facing the street. Instead of a quiet, comfortable environment conducive to sleep (even more important for someone away from their home environment), I was going to have to try to sleep in a cold, clinical environment, wired up to numerous sensors, that sounded like it was next to a freeway. NOT a good start.

It only got worse. I couldn't fall asleep, so I was allowed to use Lunesta 3, a powerful sleep aide, to get to sleep. I recall a lousy, short night of sleep with at least 1 full waking, but the study didn't really pick up much of anything. From what I hear from other people, this is not an uncommon occurrence. I have learned FAR more by collecting data with Sleep Cycle and similar apps on my phone and tablet at home and, more importantly, have been able to collect much more data and apply corrections based on it.

As such, I have the following feelings about sleep studies:

1) They are only effective when the sleep environment is perfect – this means quiet, comfortable, proper temperature, and run by experts. At the very least, it must be equal to your normal home environment.

2) Whenever possible, a sleep study should be done in the home as opposed to in a facility. In recent years, it has become possible to have equipment loaned to you to use at home after being shown how to connect it all up and use it. This is a HUGE improvement over trying to fall asleep in a hospital lab with sleep deprived third shift lab personnel watching over you. You also can generally use the equipment for a week or more to get a larger, more accurate sampling. This method has significantly lower cost and delivers much more accurate data – a win/win. Part of the reason for my personal success in improving my sleep is the sheer volume of data I have collected and been able to utilize in the optimal sleep environment – my home.

So, if you are thinking about having an expensive sleep study that is not covered by insurance, I strongly suggest you first monitor your sleep at home with the inexpensive tools we have discussed here. At a very minimum, the data could give your doctor a guide into where to look. In my most recent major sleep disturbance which required surgical correction, I discovered the issue and cause myself using tools I describe in this book. Being aware and active in your own sleep evaluation and treatment is a very worthwhile endeavor.

Interesting Discoveries from My Early Sleep Metrics

Very early on in my collection of sleep metrics, I noticed some extremely interesting patterns that have held up over time. By noticing these patterns, I was able to exploit them to improve my sleep. I believe they will apply to the vast majority of others, so here they are.

Interesting Correlation 1

In the first correlation, note the parallel divergence of the graph lines around March to May. The later I went to bed, the worse my sleep quality became. When I saw this pattern, I began making a concerted effort to get to bed on time. Instead of an alarm to wake up, I now have a reminder set in my phone to help me get to bed on time. It first reminds me at 9:30 and then again at 10:30. As a result over the past 5 years, my average bedtime has become no later than 11:30 PM (and still falling) and my regularity – the consistency of my getting to bed at this time which is a feature Sleep Cycle began tracking a year or so ago – is around 90%. These things are definitely helpful in maintaining a proper circadian cycle and improving sleep both short and long term.

Interesting Correlation

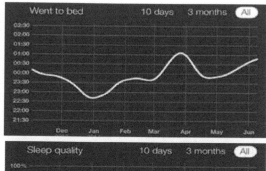

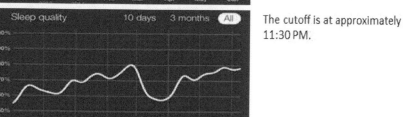

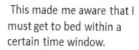

As time to bed got later, sleep quality decreased proportionately.

This made me aware that I must get to bed within a certain time window.

The cutoff is at approximately 11:30 PM.

As you can see, as my bed time got later beyond 11:30 PM, my night's sleep quality immediately diminished. What's more, as I got my bedtime headed back towards that 11:30 baseline, my sleep quality went right back up. This is a powerful illustration of the importance of keeping a regular bedtime in the optimal range for your particular situation. In sleep research this phenomenon is known as "regularity" and is now tracked by Sleep Cycle.

Interesting Correlation 2

The next interesting correlation I rapidly discovered is certainly linked to the time I get to bed, which is the overall time in bed I spend each night. In a very similar manner to the first correlation, when my time in bed went below a specific duration, my sleep quality diminished.

Interesting Correlation #2

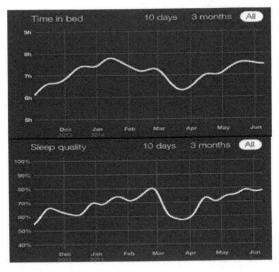

Over time, I also noticed a direct correlation between time in bed and sleep quality. For me, 7+ hours is necessary for the best sleep quality.

As you can see, when my time in bed goes below 7 hours as it does where the dip begins in March here, sleep quality drops off proportionately. When I increased time in bed, sleep quality went right back up proportionately. Over time this has shown me that I need 7.5 to 8.5 hours in bed to get sufficient sleep quality each night.

These are extremely important things to be aware of. By using a reminder to get to bed at a proper time, and dedicating the ensuing hours to sleeping until an appropriate wake up time range, you should not need an alarm to wake and should be able to get a quality night's sleep. Becoming aware of these things is a major part of the battle - I really had no idea prior to tracking these details.

Contiguous Sleep

Back in 2005 when I first began looking into my sleep, I NEVER slept an entire night all the way through before that one magical night that lead to my research. I would guess that 1-3 awakenings were the norm for me, and I also suspect that is true for a lot of you reading this.

One of the major things I believed was causing this was a need to urinate a least once a night, which is a common thing I hear from people over age 30 and especially from men. The general belief is that we wake up because we need to urinate, however I have come to believe that the actual situation is that we have to urinate because we wake up. Before I explain this, let me say that I am assuming that, like myself, you have no urinary disorders or other contributing factors. In men this generally means a healthy prostate and related systems.

Consider your bladder: it is a watertight vessel that is made of flexible material similar to rubber. Indeed, the word bladder has come to mean a flexible container for holding liquids in most contexts. Like the stomach and other organs which are flexible and hold variable content volumes, the bladder is subject to conditioning. It's maximum volume can be influenced over the long term by stretching to hold larger volumes or by frequent emptying to shrink its general size. This is not something that we normally do in a conscious manner. Under normal conditions, we all would sleep 7+ hours contiguously every night and our bladder would be receiving its longest period of volume conditioning during this time. Once we damage our sleep and start waking up and relieving ourselves, we perceive that we awake because we have to go, but that is not necessarily the case.

When I formed this theory, I began putting it to the test. If I fully awakened during the night, I would always attempt to go back to sleep immediately and only relieve myself if I felt an urgent need. This is what I do to this day. In my early days of sleep metrics, I rarely slept contiguously through the entire night and my overall bladder capacity was poor. Today I sleep all the way through the night more often than not (approximately 90% of nights) and relieving myself is often not even the first thing I do upon waking in the AM. I have gone over the years from waking up and urinating 1-3 times a night to sleeping all night and waiting 8+ hours to go every night. I will admit that, on occasion, I do awake in the morning from a dream in which I need to go and am looking for a restroom! But other than that, there has not been any issue. This is a re-training that takes a long time and can only be achieved once your sleep issues are resolved, but I have done it and so can you. A physician's input is a wise choice on this matter if that is not obvious.

Waking up once per night is not an unusual nor necessarily bad thing. In fact, there is considerable research and historical reference to "second sleep" or bi-phasic sleep. As I understand it, this was a common pattern where people went to bed sometime after sunset and would routinely awaken around midnight. Sometimes they would eat or do something, but then always go back to sleep thereafter. This has led many who study sleep to think this might be a normally occurring phenomenon, but the jury is still out.

Once in a great while this happens to me and I get up and do something briefly then head back to sleep. But the longer I have focused on my sleep, the rarer this has become. All my best sleep scores and most refreshing results have come from nights during which I experienced 7+ hours of contiguous sleep, so that is what I strive for. If I wake up, I try to immediately go back to sleep. I am now generally successful in doing this, even if I feel a slight need to urinate. It is all about conditioning yourself. In my opinion, people who indulge or condition themselves into becoming "night owls" in any regular manner develop major sleep issues and are some of the worst about conning themselves into believing it is normal or works for them. Without exception, human beings ae designed to sleep at night, all night.

This reconditioning will take you time to achieve — months to years. I saw improvements in weeks to months and my first few nights of contiguous sleep were pretty thrilling and gave me a real feeling of improvement. Give yourself time and use metrics consistently to keep track. It took you a long time to unwittingly condition yourself for bad sleep so re-conditioning yourself for good sleep will take time as well. Time and consistency are the keys to success, and each increment of success builds the foundation for further improvement. The fact that I am still improving after 7+ years of collecting data is a perfect example of this. I can tell you this: once your sleep starts improving, getting to sleep every night and seeing how much better you can do becomes a bit of a compulsion — a good one. Friends I have helped often send me 100% sleep charts in the morning with a sense of pride in the message containing them. One even thanked me for "gamifying" sleep improvement.

Breathing: Priority 1

Now that you have learned the history of how we all destroyed our own sleep and have equipped yourself with sleep monitoring metrics to gather data, I can tell you the absolute most important thing to experience proper sleep: breathing.

As a scientist by nature and profession, I immediately set out analyzing what had happened after my date night with recreational drug use back in 2005 that lead to that blissful night of sleep. I figured it out in a matter of days.

One of the interesting things about cocaine, in its pure form, is that it is a very effective vasoconstrictor. That is to say, it shrinks the blood vessels it comes into contact with thus reducing circulatory blood flow to the local area where it was administered. This is a large part of the reason that it has anesthetic properties – the reduced blood flow also reduces sensation in the area (like cutting off circulation by lying on your arm and having it go numb). That is why cocaine is used to this very day in some types of surgery – it can numb an area and reduce blood flow – perfect for surgical work in some cases. The patient feels little and blood is minimal in the surgical field for the surgeon so he can see what he needs to.

I had always noticed that nasally ingesting cocaine would lead, at least initially, to my nose opening up to breathe easier to some degree. It wasn't generally obvious because it is masked in large part by the anesthetic effect – you feel less, so it's hard to notice any improved airflow. If you are a "normal" person who can always breathe 100% through your nose, you'd likely notice little change.

So now I was on to something: it appeared that cocaine had made it easier to breathe through my nose resulting in better sleep despite the stimulant effect of the drug itself. Apparently, breathing was so critical to sleep that it could compensate for even one of the strongest stimulants known, cocaine, and allow for a good night's sleep on top of it. While the alcohol I'd ingested undoubtedly contributed as well by offsetting the stimulant effects somewhat, I was pretty sure I was on to something. One thing seemed clear to me: *my breathing wasn't as good as other people's and definitely not as good as it should be.* It made sense: all my life, I couldn't stand to hear my own voice when it was recorded – it had an awful, nasal sound to it – think of Nicolas Cage or James Gandolfini. It was like I was holding my nose pinched shut while talking. Other people didn't sound that way, at least not from my observation. But my father sounded that way and, as a kid, I could hear him snoring sometimes on a different level of the house through a closed door. Come to think of it, my sisters and my mother also had that nasal quality to their voices, and I could remember all of them snoring at some point in their lives (when young in the case of my sisters – under 18). I also knew I snored at least sometimes from catching myself on occasion and also from girlfriends who told me so. I was clearly beginning to unearth something here.

Note: it is interesting to note that James Gandolfini, better known as Tony Soprano and one of the greatest actors of our time, died at age 51 of heart disease. I was often struck during the countless hours I spent watching and re-watching his brilliant performances in **The Sopranos** by his terribly nasal voice and labored breathing that was often audible even in the edited final sound. (Breathing noises by an actor are usually edited out if not there for a reason in a scene.) Gandolfini was significantly overweight for his height and I would wager very good money that he had severe sleep issues which caused or contributed to his heart disease and subsequent untimely death at age 51. It was painful for me to listen to his breathing/speaking at times. This was a man with serious breathing difficulties and almost certainly sleep issues.

I began a series of loosely controlled experiments. Clearly, cocaine was NOT something I wanted to use for these, so I looked into both other means of vasoconstricting the nasal passages and generally improving breathing. I quickly discovered that anything that would open up the nasal passages by vasoconstriction would, indeed, allow for greatly improved breathing and sleep. Unfortunately, I also discovered that ANY such vasoconstrictor that does this will also cause what is known as a "rebound" effect.

Most who have used cocaine intranasally know that about 12 hours later their nose will become very congested and hard to breathe through – that is rebound effect; the substance which shrinks the blood vessels and tissues in the nose wears off and then when they return to normal they first swell past normal and then reduce down to normal state. I recalled a guy I'd known in college who would take decongestant the morning after using cocaine to mitigate this issue. I had the same results with all vasoconstrictors, so I am going to save you the trouble of even bothering with them. I had done some testing of other nasal decongestants to try to recreate the effect I'd gotten from cocaine, but any over the counter medication I found also had a stimulant effect causing sleep to actually suffer rather than improve and also exhibited a rebound effect 24 hours later. As such, I do not generally recommend using any nasal decongestant spray for improving breathing during sleep, not even as an experiment. I will discuss various breathing aides that can be used to help you test improving nasal breathing when you sleep. Until then, the first thing I want you to know is this: breathing is the number one most critical thing involved in getting a good night's sleep, period. If you remember only one thing from his book, that should be it. Breathing is EVERYTHING when it comes to sleep. If you are not able to breathe properly (and we will discuss what that means) nothing else will improve your sleep significantly. Everything else we will cover is secondary to that so, if you have a known breathing issue, I implore you to go immediately to work to resolve it. Just remember: when it comes to sleep, breathing is **everything.**

Proper Sleep Breathing

Something I came to understand but nobody ever told me is that there is a right way to breathe during sleep: 100% nasally. Breathing through your mouth while asleep indicates a real problem. I never knew this and probably breathed orally while asleep most of my life from my early 20s until my early 40s.

Without proper breathing, you might sleep, but you will not get proper sleep, and that is the case for a great many people who wake up tired every day. The point of sleep is that it is *restorative* to a myriad of physical and neural processes. If you're not getting the proper kind of sleep in the necessary quantity, you will stay alive, but the quality of your life and its length will continually deteriorate – at a far faster rate than nature intended. Look at your dog, your cat, or just about any other land animal on Earth – they all sleep. What's more, they all sleep properly and in sufficient quantities. Your dog doesn't push himself to go 2 days without sleeping and your cat might sleep up to 20 hours a day. They innately obey the natural laws of circadian cycle and sleep when they feel the need and/or at night (cats are nocturnal hunters, so they like to sleep a bit more during the day)

There's something else which, if you watch them sleep, you will notice about your pets: they breathe properly when they sleep. That is to say their mouth is normally completely closed and they are breathing 100% through their nose. What you do during waking hours carries over into sleep. Any opportunity for mouth breathing inhaling or exhaling will increase the chances of mouth breathing during sleep. Hospital studies have established that nocturnal mouth breathing is a primary cause of loud snoring. Snoring is an indicator of sleep apnea, and sleep apnea is a precursor to stroke, diabetes, heart disease and early death. In studies of patients with congestive heart failure run over a decade, the death rate of patients with sleep apnea who did not accept CPAP treatment was twice as high as those who did. But the major finding of the same study was that in persons with sleep apnea the risk of stroke is 3-4 times as great as in those without sleep apnea. [9]

Is that a surprise to you to hear? Did you not know that you should be breathing 100% nasally when sleeping? It was a surprise to me, and how I came to learn it is a long and fascinating story that will explain a lot.

---

[9] National Geographic Naked Science: Dead Tired

Proper breathing during sleep is done 100% through the nose. This is something that nobody, for the most part, ever tells us. Probably because most people don't know it. Most of us have seen many animals that breathe air when they are asleep and, with few exceptions, you will nearly always see them breathe entirely nasally while asleep. Dogs are a great example. (It should be noted that some breeds engineered to have shortened faces and snouts, like pugs or bulldogs, have been made to generally have terrible breathing issues as a result of this selective breeding and do not generally apply in this example) I have observed dogs of mine sleeping countless hours and the vast majority of that time they were breathing nasally. Occasionally their position or something else would make them snore or breathe orally, but that was the exception. Breathing nasally during sleep is the way that works best. Once I learned this, I had to re-train myself to do it by default.

Additionally, mouth breathing causes a number of additional issues when sleeping. When breathing orally, we lose up to 40% more water through vapor in our breath dehydrating us while asleep. I always noticed I was significantly more dried out and thirsty upon waking when I breathed orally overnight. Worse still, the drying out of the mouth and throat leads to issues with breath, gums and teeth and causes throat irritation from the dryness. These factors can contribute to a host of secondary problems as a result.

So, do you breathe properly when you are asleep? Well, you're asleep, so you probably don't know. Just because you start out your night of sleep breathing nasally doesn't mean you continue that way. Here's a quick test: take a few full breaths in and out breathing through your mouth. Because the size of your mouth is vastly larger than your nasal openings, you can take in the greatest volume of air with the least resistance through your mouth. This is why, when you become fatigued or oxygen deprived during exercise, you will naturally switch to mouth or combined mouth/nose breathing: oral breathing allows the greatest volume of oxygen into your system the fastest. Now, take an equal number of breaths in and out only through your nose. Do you feel a difference in airflow? In an ideal situation, when not exercising, your ability to move air through your nose should feel 100% or nearly 100% of the flow you have through your mouth. If it is less, try this a few times and then see where you think your nasal breathing capacity compares to your oral breathing capacity. Consider your mouth breathing flow to be a 10 on a scale of 1 to 10. Then, ask yourself what you think your nasal breathing rates on the same scale. The intake capacity of your mouth is greater than your nose, and there are far fewer turns and obstructions between it and the portion of your airway that it shares with your nose, so oral breathing is always going to have a better capacity to move more air faster than nasal. However, your nasal air capacity should feel pretty close to your oral capacity. I'd say around 80 to 85%. Ask yourself, if your best oral breathing is a 10, what number is your best nasal breathing? They should be this close. If they are not, it is likely you may have an issue breathing through your nose. If it is a 7 or less (i.e.; 70% or less of the airflow you get through your mouth), then there is a very good chance you have an issue. Try this many times under different conditions – early morning, before bed, when you wake up in the middle of the night, midday, etc. What is your average nasal airflow percentage? Most importantly, try it after you've been lying down for a while. When you are standing, fluid in your body is drawn away from your head at all times by gravity. When you are lying down, it can move to put more pressure into your head – you've probably experienced this in an uncomfortable fashion when trying to sleep with a head cold. (Interestingly, astronauts in zero G for extended periods have trouble discerning when they are thirsty because gravity is not present to draw fluid downward away from their head giving the normally recognized indications of dry mouth, etc.) It is not uncommon for nasal breathing capacity to be lower when lying down than standing, so get a good idea of your lying nasal airflow and see how it compares to your oral airflow. Generally speaking, a 7 out of 10 or lower is indication that improvement may be needed and that breathing is impacting your sleep. I routinely experience nasal airflow 20% worse lying down than when standing up and often can only breathe through one or the other side of my nose while in a lying position – clearly an issue.

It is also of value to block each side of your nose with your thumb and test whether or not your breathing capacity feels equal in both sides of your nose. It is not uncommon for the airflow to be slightly different, but if one side is significantly better than the other this is something you will want to have checked out by a doctor – an ENT specialist (otolaryngologist). For many years I experienced variability in my nasal breathing where only one side or the other was generally clear to breathe through – this was obviously a huge negative factor in proper sleep in addition to a problem with normal breathing and blood oxygenation during the day.

When you are lying down, fluid distribution and other factors affect your airway and oral/nasal breathing capabilities, so you will also want to try these tests while lying in bed. If you determine that your nasal airflow is significantly lower than oral airflow or that your nasal airflow is not balanced from any of these simple tests, these are matters to take up with a medical professional and resolve before proceeding. This was what I first had to do.

I became aware after my one night of fantastic sleep that I was unable to breathe much, if at all, through my nose. Having first had success (if entirely accidentally) with a chemical vasoconstrictor of the illegal variety, I decided to try some experiments with another chemical vasoconstrictor – a legal one. The medication was oxymetazoline –better known as Afrin, though it is generically available under many different names. Using oxymetazoline inhalant mist, I was able to duplicate the free breathing and good sleep that I had experienced previously. I now knew I was on to something. Free nasal breathing, at least for me, lead to good sleep.

However, there was a problem; oxymetazoline is a *dangerous* medicine. It is one of those compounds that, when you know what it can do, makes you really wonder why it is available over the counter – it probably shouldn't be. The first problem is that about 24 hours after using Oxymetazoline the free breathing comes to an end and there is a "rebound" or refractory period for most people during which your nose becomes *far more* blocked than it was before you took the medicine. For me, this lasted several hours. There is a trap here in that many people, experiencing this stuffiness after clear breathing, will take another dose of the medication to counteract it. This can quickly lead to a vicious cycle where the user takes the medicine with increasing frequency trying just to get back to normal breathing again. But, it's a lot worse than that because oxymetazoline, if taken more than twice in 24 hours, seems to accumulate in the bloodstream and has a nasty side effect – acute anxiety. There are recorded cases of people taking too much of the drug for a 1-2 week period and being so overwhelmed by the anxiety that they *committed suicide*. This stuff is not to be trifled with whatsoever. I personally experienced this incredibly unpleasant level of toxicity on more than one occasion and would not EVER want to experience it again. There is significant medical literature indicating that oxymetazoline can cause or trigger stimulant induced psychosis (!) when used for an extended period.[10] So please, pay close attention to my next sentence: If you use Oxymetazoline for a 1 or 2 night (maximum!) test, throw it away after that.

It offers NO safe, long term solutions for improving nasal breathing, only a good test for determining if you have an issue. If you find you have trouble breathing nasally you can try it for ONE night to confirm that you may sleep better if you can breathe through your nose, then it's time to see a doctor for a proper solution. A CPAP machine will give you an immediate fix until a permanent surgical or other one can be made.

[10] Brian Ticoll, MD, CCFP; Gerald Shugar, MD, FRCP, "Paranoid Psychosis Induced By Oxymetazoline Nasal Spray," Feb 1, 1994

If you can breathe well through your nose, the next thing to determine is if you are breathing properly at night – with your mouth closed and entirely through your nose. If you are able to breathe well nasally, or if, like me, you had surgery to make this possible and now need to break old habits, there is a technique covered in the non-surgical breathing aides ahead known as mouth taping which will help you to develop this habit. The other tactics in that section can help significantly improve your nasal breathing if it is not bad enough to require surgery but still needs improving. I use several of them on an ongoing basis.

Snoring: The Sound of Gradual Death

Of all the things I can think of in our lives today that are major health risks that we ignore or take too lightly, snoring is number one.

Wherever we might see snoring depicted in popular culture, it is shown as something quite different than what it really is. I think my first awareness of snoring was in cartoons when I was a kid of maybe age 3 or 4. Whenever someone was asleep, this would be indicated by loud, whimsical snoring. Sometimes the sound would be imaged as sawing wood and I recall that being an old colloquialism for sleep – referring to a time during which I'd been asleep, my dad would laughingly say, "You were sawing wood". (Though at that age I doubt I snored, but that was just a common way of describing sleep which speaks to how common snoring must have been.)

Wherever snoring appears in popular culture, it is depicted as something common, normal, whimsical, indicative of someone sleeping soundly. None of these things could be further from the truth. Snoring is the sound of an obstructed airway partially (and sometimes totally) choking off the air supply of someone trying to sleep. There is nothing lighthearted nor anything whimsical about it; it is the sound of medical distress and, ultimately, a long, slow death. We need to change how we view this phenomenon.

I have had to deal with chronic snoring twice now in my 15-year journey to better sleep. In the early days, I suffered from a combination of throat and nasal issues all of which required surgical correction: A deviated septum, enlarged nasal turbinates, vibrating soft palate tissues, and diminished nasal passage capacity. These things have an interactive synergy that combine to make breathing far worse than any one alone. After my surgery, I no longer snored and could sleep through the night breathing through my nose after using the taping method to train myself not to breathe through my mouth, over the course of about a year. Things were looking up.

Then, a few years later in mid-2017, I got a shock. I had an increasing number of nights where my sleep quality seemed to go bad during the night. I was not sure what changed, but the data was shifting rapidly enough to raise alarm bells. You may recall the dip mentioned earlier in my 6-year graph in mid-2017 - this was that time. I rapidly plunged from 90% sleep quality to 70% or less:

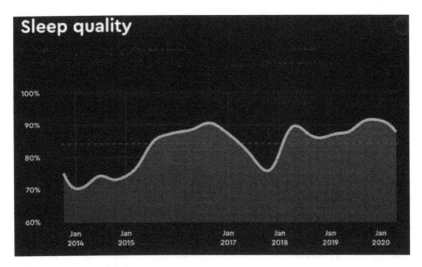

Snoring beginning again in 2017 derailed my ongoing progress.

Back then, Sleep Cycle did not detect and record/log snoring so I used a different method. I took a video camera with night vision and set it up to record myself in bed asleep all night. It only took one night to get a nasty surprise: I was snoring again, worse than ever and at times struggling for air. I had a serious problem. Sometime later in 2017, Sleep Cycle added this functionality and I started getting detailed data about my snoring. Not only was it a problem, it was a growing problem and I was heading into a dangerous place very fast. I began seeking medical assistance and compiling the data from Sleep Cycle to show the doctors I met with. By December of 2017, my average nightly snore time had increased to over an hour and 30 minutes:

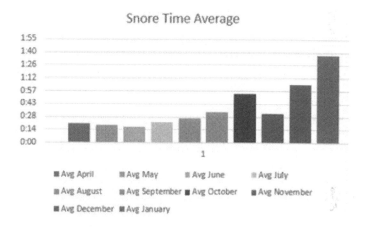

My rapidly increasing snore times graphed in 2017.

I was in serious trouble and I knew it. This was not survivable without some kind of intervention. I felt like I had back in 2006, and that was incredibly bad. I immediately began seeking medical assistance. Only now would I discover just how unprepared even the best doctors can be when it comes to snoring.

I first went to my dentist, who I had known for over 15 years and is a top-notch DDS. I know that because my own father was a dentist and my mother and sisters were his assistants growing up. His dental office was quite literally in our house for years, so I grew up in it. When I found my dentist in Los Angeles, I had done a lot of research in order to find him and was very happy with my discovery. He was the best and cutting edge…. but not for snoring.

He made me a jaw positioner based on the only real treatment option he apparently knew at the time. When I first used it, it seemed to work… until it didn't. After a week or two, I was right back to snoring and a few hundred dollars poorer. I then looked into the dentist Joe Rogan had mentioned and learned he had patented some interesting types of mouthpieces for snoring remediation and wondered if that might be the cure for me. The patents were interesting and used a completely different methodology than my dentist's aligner had. As I previously mentioned, $3000 later I threw the device, which made things only worse, in the trash.

At this point, I was becoming desperate and I realized I was going to most likely have to solve this problem myself somehow. One of the things that I feel makes me better than most at my job in computer and network security is that I *never* guess at the cause of a problem and just throw possible solutions at it – I always use diagnostic tools and techniques until I *know* what I am dealing with and then can apply a well-considered solution. I drilled down on the facts I had: Something had changed in early 2017 to cause my snoring. I had seen two medical practitioners, and neither had resolved the issue. It seemed to me that they had just thrown cures at my problem without knowing exactly what had caused it. That seemed to be the key issue: WHY was I snoring – what was the physical cause? I thought long and hard about this and came up with an experiment that I thought might help me determine the cause.

In my work I pride myself on being extremely thorough – more than most people in the same field. I can secure systems because I can know or build every inch of them. In order to provide the highest level of security for clients, we sometimes even wire their buildings and homes ourselves to make sure it is done correctly. People who come to work for me learn first elemental tasks like how to make data cables from scratch so they too can know every inch of a system.

Sometimes, we need to get a cable through a place we cannot see, or look for damage or a tapped line in such a place, such as inside a wall. In the past several years, this has been made much easier by the availability of low-cost fiber optic endoscopes – similar in many ways to those used by surgeons in arthroscopic surgeries. For under $100, today anyone can buy a full color, lighted fiber scope with magnification that will display on the screen of their phone or tablet. When we need to see inside a wall or such to do our work, we slip one in and look around.

When I snored, I could feel it in my throat, so I reasoned that if I took my (sterilized) fiber optic scope and put it in my mouth and made myself snore, I might be able to see what was going on. In under 30 seconds, I had the answer.

For whatever reason, my uvula – the fleshy structure that hangs down from above at the back of the throat, was obstructing my airway and causing me to snore. I made an appointment to see my ENT who had done the surgeries on me years earlier and went to see him. I told him what was going on, showed him my months long collection of snoring data showing the increasing issue, and told him what I thought was causing my snoring. He put a different type of scope up my nose and through my sinus cavity and down the back of my throat to view the same area from behind and confirmed what I had thought: my uvula was obstructing my airway.

The takeaway here is what I now know and you will benefit from if you snore: NEVER accept any treatment for snoring until you know WHY you are snoring. How I got through seeing two medical providers who gave me solutions without actually discerning the cause of the problem is beyond me, but it should never have happened. The very first thing they should have done, in my opinion, was to ask me to try to make myself snore while somehow observing what took place. It is egregious for a medical practitioner to apply a treatment without even attempting to witness and identify the exact problem. Before accepting or paying for any treatment for snoring, do whatever you need to in order to find out the EXACT cause. My life experience has taught me that 80-90 %+ of the people in any field are mediocre to bad at best so one has to work hard to find the 10% or less who are really good. Despite our societal deification of medical practitioners, they are no different. Screen your physicians thoroughly and extensively, and go to the right practitioner for the issue you need help with.

After determining the cause of my new snoring problem, I began contemplating a correction. I could simply get surgery asap, but that was a real disruption to my life and, before I did it, I wanted to know why this had happened. I also needed some kind of an immediate fix because I felt like I was dying and would not last long snoring 90+ minutes per night. I was back to feeling how I had years earlier when I was absolutely miserable and not sure I could continue. I needed relief fast.

Once again, I decided to help myself. I knew that a Continuous Positive Airway Pressure device might be able to resolve the issue right away to buy me some time until I could have surgery. Eschewing medical help for the time, I did my own research and bought one online and learned all I needed to use and program it. (Note: this is a questionable/gray area as many places will not sell CPAPs without a medical prescription and others will. The fact is, however, that anyone can generally get one and it is well within the capabilities of many people to use without a physician. The average biohacker would not even blink at this, but be aware that for the average person a physician's help is a better option.) Within 2 days, I slept using a nasal CPAP unit and had a perfect night with zero snoring. As you can see from the graph, by January of 2019 I was back to normal. The CPAP had bought me the time to carefully consider my surgical options and allowed me to get back to normal sleep in the interim. I still use it nightly while I compare best surgical options for uvular reduction and wait for hospitals to be open for elective surgeries again during COVID-19. I really look forward to not needing it anymore even as thankful as I am for the relief it has provided. CPAP and similar devices provide relief, but do not resolve underlying issues. To me, fixing the underlying issue is always the best option once that can be done.

Within a few months, I had determined what likely caused my new snoring problem. Since my mid-30s, I have done experimentation and research into athletic performance enhancing medications and techniques. These have included a number of anabolic compounds including testosterone, which always gave me good results with little to no downsides. In late 2016, I had started feeling sluggish and lethargic and, as I had done many times through the years in conjunction with my biohacking experiments, went to a lab to have blood drawn to look at my levels. I noticed that my testosterone was in the low end of the range, which was common for my age at that time, and decided to begin testosterone replacement therapy (TRT). The results were good and I have continued ever since. There are always some possible side effects when taking exogenous testosterone and these effects are different for different age ranges and different individuals. Lo and behold, I learned that enlargement of the uvula is a known, reported side effect of TRT. So now I knew the likely cause. It made perfect sense. Since I did not want to go off of TRT and will likely continue it the rest of my life, I decided to pursue a surgical reduction of my uvula. As of this writing I have not done it yet, but as soon as COVID-19 allows, I will do so.

Let my odyssey be a lesson: If you find from Sleep Cycle or other means that you have a snoring issue, find out *exactly* why and then look into the possible treatment options. Save yourself a lot of time, money, and potential downsides.

Above all, understand that snoring is a warning signal and take it very seriously. Snoring tends to start in our 20s and only gets worse as we age if not corrected. Take a look at this data collected globally by Sleep Cycle which supports this:

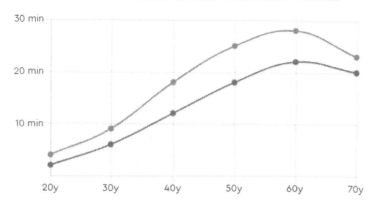

Snoring average by age demographic worldwide. [11]

Over ten years, 37.4 million people have downloaded Sleep Cycle and it has tracked 4.38 billion hours of sleep. (500,000 years' worth). This includes *131.4 million hours of snoring* – that's 15,000 years. And remember, snoring has only been tracked since 2017. That is an alarming statistic that we should take close note of.

---

[11] From Sleep Cycle www.sleepcycle.com

Breathing Aides for Sleep – Non-Surgical

Opening up the nasal airway to allow proper breathing is not something that can only be accomplished surgically. In fact, some of the best improvements I have ever received (even better than surgical) have come from the methods I am about to describe. I use them on an ongoing basis in combinations with great success. You can try them immediately for comparatively little or no cost and get an idea of how much better you will sleep when you can breathe freely.

Breathe Right Strips

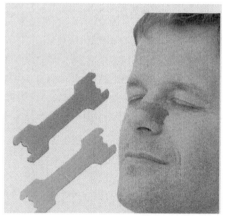

Perhaps the best known non-surgical nasal breathing aide is the Breathe Right strip. It's concept, "nasal tenting", is ingenious and simple: a springy plastic strip is adhered to the exterior of the nose midway between the bridge and the tip with strong adhesive and exerts a negative, upward force against the skin. If effectively increases the tenting effect of the nose, thereby increasing the volume of air which can flow.

These are something most people have seen at one time or another. They are used widely in some professional sports, such as football, to improve breathing and, as such, oxygen intake. The concept is simple: opening up the nasal passages more allows increased airflow. Most people feel an immediate, noticeable increase in airflow when they apply a strip. Be sure to clean the skin of your nose first (alcohol is best) to get the best adhesion. Many people use these strips long term. I personally found that the skin of my nose felt a bit sensitive after too many days/weeks in a row using them, but everyone is different. If you have issues with the adhesive pulling on your skin long term as I did, you may find the next option, nasal inserts, to be better for you long term, as I did.

Pros: Immediate result, inexpensive, works well
Cons: Visible to others (though available in minimally visible clear and flesh colors), tends to come off during sleep, long term can cause irritation to or stretching of skin, one use only disposable.

Brez Nasal Inserts

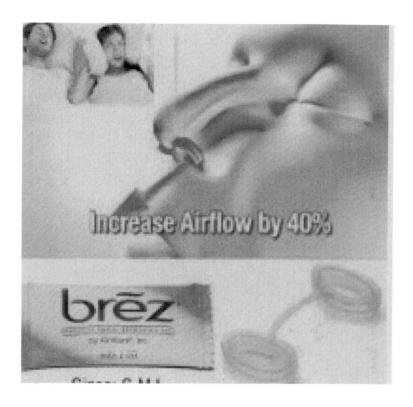

Brez and other similar nasal inserts are a very simple and incredibly effective invention. These are small tubular rubber inserts which you insert into your nostrils and in doing so impart a "tenting" effect from the inside. They come linked together by a small rubber connection, but I find it more comfortable to pull the tubes apart discarding the connector and then either use them individually or together. The reasons for this are 1) I like to sometimes use only one insert and, incidentally, you will have an easier time getting used to them using just one side initially 2) I don't need them "leashed" to get them out of my nose easily and neither will you and 3) without the connector, they are invisible in your nose, making them far less intrusive to use, especially if sleeping with another person or wearing them in public – no one will ever notice them. Sometimes, at first, it can take a bit of time to get used to having these in your nose and I recommend just doing one side at first to make this easier. Without the link between the 2 tubes, it is a bit more difficult to remove them sometimes, but your pinkie will do it. If one is giving me difficulty, I just blow that side of my nose and out it comes. There are a few similar products on the market, but Brez is the only one I have ever used and it works incredibly well. Just FYI, they can be used repeatedly for a very long time with simple cleaning – there is no need to use a new set every time unless you want to spend more money.

Pros: Immediate result, inexpensive, works well, reusable, invisible if used without link
Cons: Sometimes they get a bit out of position in the nose, but this is infrequent and easily adjusted.

Nasal Rinse

The nasal rinse is quite possibly the single most useful non-surgical breathing aide I have discovered in the last 10 years.   I had never heard of this concept until a friend who suffers from bad allergies told me about it. In the most common form, it involves the use of what is known as a Neti pot. A Neti pot is a small ceramic or plastic vessel that looks like a tea pot. There are many variations, but they generally look something like this:

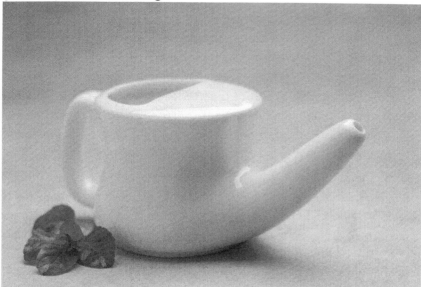

A Neti pot.

You mix saline and warm it and put it into the pot and then put the spout of the pot into one nostril with your head over a sink and turned parallel to the floor. The warm saline then goes into one side of the nose, fills the sinus cavity, and flows out the other side. This is done over a sink and the head is tilted forward and 90 degrees so that the warm water fills the sinus cavities and then flows out the opposite nostril. This is then repeated from the opposite side nostril. The result is an incredible clearing of the nasal airway and sinuses. The saline flush also removes allergens and contaminants and generally has an extremely refreshing and beneficial effect.

This takes some time to master (there are many helpful videos online) but is a lot easier to do and tolerate than it sounds. After you become proficient at it, the effect is excellent as it flushes everything out of your nose and sinuses and seems to shrink the tissues therein. It has the added benefit of greatly reducing allergy symptoms for many people and also reduces instances of sinus infection or upper respiratory infections that begin in the nasal area. My research into my own sleep has shown a significant sleep quality improvement when I have used a nasal flush and then a breathing aide, such as Brez, before sleeping. To this day I generally use a nasal flush every night.

The last time I dropped my ceramic Neti pot and broke it, I decided to replace it with a plastic squeeze bottle made for the same purpose like this one:

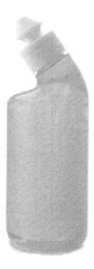

A Nasopure nasal rinse bottle.

This was a big improvement for me as I could force the fluid through my sinuses with slight pressure as opposed to waiting for it to flow with the pot, which sometimes took a while. I do not recommend using a squeeze bottle until you have first mastered the Neti Pot as I think it would have been very difficult had I not used the Neti Pot first. That being said, I find the squeeze bottle to be much superior for me.

The solution you use for nasal rinse is quite variable and bears tinkering with. Initially, I used just simple salt in the solution. (Ancient Secrets brand is my favorite) Over time, I wondered if I might add something to moisturize my nasal tissues and sinuses as I tend to experience a lot of dryness in my nose. This led to the discovery of a product called Xlear which combines salt, Xylitol (yes, the sugar substitute sweetener) and sodium bicarbonate. I noticed that the solution I made with this evacuated the sinuses much more easily and completely and also helped with moisturizing. I took to experimenting with customized mixtures and am still experimenting with them. The initial mixes have improved my sleep results 1-2 percent. Generally, I mix 3 parts Xylitol to 1 part baking soda and 1 part salt and really like the results.

In a final evolution of my nasal rinse methodology, I stumbled across a device called a Navage.

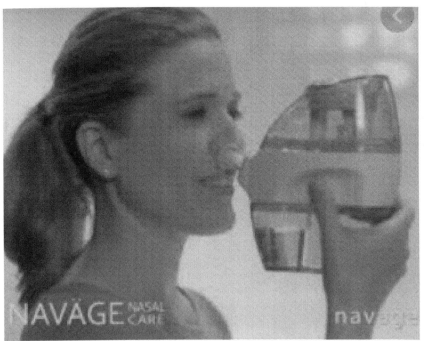

The Navage nasal rinse system.

This is perhaps the holy grail of nasal rinse systems. The Navage (Nasal Lavage) is a battery powered motorized irrigation device. It has one tank for warm saline and another to collect the used water. Soft tips plug into both sides of the nose and water is pushed out one side under force and pulled in the other with suction. After using half the water, the tips are reversed to flush the water remaining in the opposite direction. It gives the best nasal rinse of any device I have ever tried.

At around $100 the Navage is expensive, but worth it in my opinion. While it is made to use cartridges similar to a Keurig coffee maker which you must buy from the manufacturer, this can be circumvented to use your own mixtures for significantly better customization and lower cost.

Overall, my recommendation would be to use nasal rinse devices starting with the Neti pot, then the squeeze bottle, then the Navage – the order I went in was a logical progression and worked out well.

One caveat about nasal rinsing: The water MUST be warm to hot. It is surprising to find out how hot the water can be with no problem. Cold water, however, is really painful – avoid it at all costs! I warm the water – the quantity held by a Nasopure bottle - by warming it 30 seconds in my microwave. This is very effective and fast and also helps purify the water. As microwave power levels vary, test carefully when using this method. I also vary the time in summer vs winter when less/more warming is needed. Incidentally, the Nasopure bottle holds the exact amount of water needed for the Navage, so if you progress along the same path I did this makes a convenient vessel to mix and heat your solution in before pouring it into the Navage.

Pros: Effective, also helps allergies, conducive to sleep, inexpensive (other than Navage)

Cons: Somewhat of a learning curve, can feel like you have accidentally water boarded yourself if you make a mistake.

Nasal Hair Removal

I am repeatedly amazed by the immediate increase in nasal airflow I consistently get from just trimming the hair out of my nose. For the record, I do not have much nor noticeable hair in my nose, but just removing the amount that grows every week or 2 makes a VERY perceptible difference. If I had to guess how much, I'd say I easily get up to a 20% increase in airflow!

It has taken me some time to learn how to do this quickly and properly. First FORGET about using scissors or any kind of plucking. Scissors will not do an adequate job and plucking is painful and WILL cause infection, which is a nightmare. Instead, get one of the commercially available battery powered electric rotary trimmers. I use a Panasonic model which has a vacuum feature to remove the hair from the nose as it is cut.

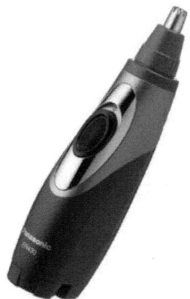

Panasonic ER430 nasal hair trimmer

To trim and remove the hair effectively, you will need to do it facing a mirror and shining a strong light into the nostril – I use a small, very bright LED flashlight. You will NOT get as good of a result doing the trimming blindly or without light – it took me a long time to learn this. Be sure to clean and oil your trimmer on a regular basis so it works well and change the cutting blades on a regular basis. Also use a fully charged battery to avoid injury. Fast and sharp is what you want.

It is just astounding to me how something seemingly so miniscule as nose hair can impede airflow, but it definitely does. If you've never done this before and have hair in your nose, you will notice a significant benefit. Beyond that, it looks a lot better than the alternative, so there's an added benefit.

Many people will make the argument that nose hair serves a purpose by diffusing incoming air, filtering out particles, and other functions that reduce sinus infections. Many physicians also support this position. However, in recent years, numerous ENTs and other physicians have come to a conclusion which I share which is that removal of nose hairs will not make any noticeable difference in your immune system to most people. My experience is that I got FAR more sinus infections before I started trimming the hair out of my nose. Indeed, when my septum was deviated and my turbinates swollen before my surgery, I reached a point where I was getting sinus infections almost weekly. Since the surgery, I've not had one infection – not one. Your results may vary, but keeping hair out of my nose and using a fairly regular nasal rinse I have not had a sinus infection in several years.

From a technical point of view, mucous in the nostrils can capture and stop further inhalation of debris, particles, and bacteria. The nostril hairs increase the effectiveness of this by providing more surface area for the mucous to cling to and, in doing so, creating more of a "filter" in the nose. After removing this hair from my nose for many years I cannot discern any difference in this filtering capacity. Your mileage may vary, but probably won't. If one is in a dusty environment, they should be using a mask, not relying on nasal hair.

The one thing doctors on both sides of the issue DO agree about is that you should NOT pluck hairs from the nose, ever. Plucking is far more likely to cause infection or, equally bad, ingrown hairs, which are very painful inside the nose and prone to infection as well.

I have done research into the possibility of permanent nose hair removal by laser. While I am still looking into this, it looks like a very promising possible future solution that I may very well try. My experience is that nasal hair serves no valuable function and impedes airflow into the nose. As such, I can do without it entirely.

Pros: Easy, effective, aesthetically preferable
Cons: None that I am aware of. Laser removal is painful I am told.

Mouth Taping

If someone had told me about this method of breathing improvement before I stumbled onto it, I'd have looked at them like they were insane.

Before I explain this technique and teach you how to try it, I want to make it very clear that 1) you need to have a nasal breathing capacity of at least 70% of your oral breathing capacity (Refer back to earlier in the book when we tested this and, if you didn't do the test, do it now) and 2) you should have experimented with all the other nasal breathing improvement techniques to get optimal nasal breathing before trying this. Most nights, I cannot use this method without performing a nasal rinse and using an airway increasing aide (usually Brez) in at least one nostril.

Once you have your nasal breathing at an acceptable level, you can give mouth taping a try. I really had not expected the improvements I got from this technique when I first thought about it and looked up. Much to my surprise, I learned that there were a good many people who had experimented with this technique and I benefitted from their work. The result is a technique from which I got, on average, a 10% sleep quality improvement.

Keeping your mouth closed during sleep has a number of benefits. You dry out less because you do not exhale nearly as much humid air as when you breathe nasally. Snoring is greatly diminished because the airway is in a more functional position. And since the mouth is sealed, air pressure and flow through the nostrils is maximized. These factors combined make a real difference. I believe tongue posture is partially involved in this improvement – that is discussed next.

Before describing how to do this, I want to make something very clear: what we are doing here is making your mouth stay closed, NOT sealing it from getting any air. Under NO circumstances should you ever do that for sleeping – it could conceivably have fatal results. Do not even think about it. You want to be able to get air through your mouth if you need to do so during the night due to a change in nasal breathing capacity, such as might be caused by a position change. What we are doing is two things: 1) closing your mouth so you will breathe automatically through your nose and 2) helping your mouth to seal, since it is prone to moisture loss, so as to keep you from losing hydration while you are asleep. This is one of those things I spoke about in the disclaimer at the very beginning of this book that you should check with a doctor before trying. Please be very careful.

I am told by many people that they have been able to achieve the same effect using a mouthpiece created by a dentist or from another source. I believe this is the case for some people. For me, however, I tend to feel less comfortable using such a jaw positioning mouthpiece and it seems unnecessary.

The technique for mouth taping is simple. First, you will need some surgical tape which you can get at any drug store or from online sources. I like to use the 3M Micropore 1-inch tape. The reasons I have come to like this tape (by no means am I averse to trying others if you find a particularly good one) is mainly that, because it is paper based, it is not too strong while having extremely good adhesion. I usually make the adhesive a bit weaker by sticking it to the palm of my hand and pulling it off once or twice so that it won't be too hard to remove in the morning. Surgical tapes adhere to skin VERY well for days and you don't want to abrade yourself or hurt your skin when you remove it, so be careful.

Here's how to apply the tape: Cut a piece about 1 to 1.5 inches long. You can fine tune this length over time – shorter if there's too much adhesion, longer if you need more. Place the tape vertically starting under your nose across both lips of your closed mouth and ending just below your bottom lip and above your chin like this:

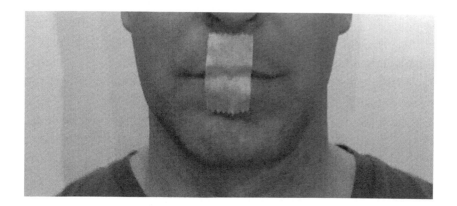

At first this might seem a bit concerning and cause you to worry about getting air via your mouth should you need to. I had this very same concern the minute I tried this. However, it is a simple matter to get air or even drink water if you need to through the open sides of your mouth. You can easily open one or both sides next to the tape anytime you need to like this:

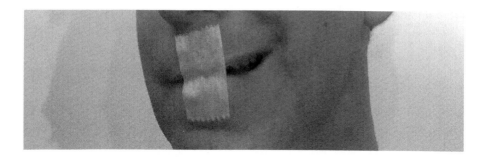

When you are sleeping, if you need to you will be able to do this just as easily. I have logged more than 300 nights using this technique with never any issue whatsoever. Indeed, this simple technique works so well that I immediately started using it every night. The purpose of the tape is really about mouth and jaw being held in a closed position, not sealing your mouth as an airway. When your mouth is open, you naturally stop breathing through your nose and when your mouth is closed, you do the opposite. Keeping your mouth closed helps condition you to breathe nasally during sleep and get back to proper breathing.

It was my hope that, after some extended period of using this technique, keeping my mouth closed would become automatic and nasal breathing would become my automatic norm. In fact, that is exactly what did happen and now I no longer need to use it.

One minor issue of this technique is that if you wake up and need to drink some water, as I often do, it can be a bit challenging. I used to keep water by my bed in a common screw top water bottle but now, since I began this taping technique, I use a sports type bottle with built in straw instead and this makes it a lot easier. Additionally, I believe in minimizing the time I am awake if I do wake up at night and also minimizing the mental tasks that might serve to awaken me further, such as unscrewing a bottle top and then re-closing it. (this is a very simple task, but at 4AM it is enough to start tipping the scale against your falling back to sleep easily after a quick drink.) Drinking from the bottle with the straw makes the entire process faster and simpler even with my mouth taped, which is overall a big advantage for improving my sleep. I don't even need to open my eyes.

Again, be VERY careful and patient when removing the tape. If you pull it off too quickly or not at a proper angle, you can easily get red abrasion marks like this:

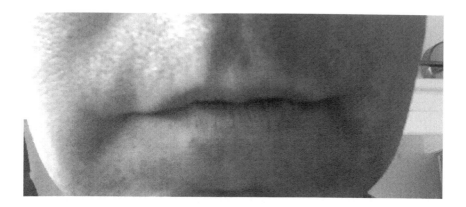

These minor abrasions will go away in a day or two, but it's still no fun to have them. Also, do NOT put tape over an injured area again until it has healed! Shift the tape to one side or the other or take a night or two off until the affected area has completely healed.

If the tape is extremely strong or difficult to remove, a bit of alcohol or mineral spirits on a cotton swab can help to safely remove it quickly. Again, sticking the tape to the palm of your hand two or three times before putting it in place can be very helpful in preventing this issue.

Tongue Posture

Tongue posture is something I only first heard of in the last year but likely I have benefitted from via mouth taping and/or proper sleep breathing unknowingly for some time.

Tongue Posture simply refers to what is considered the best/correct position for your tongue when your mouth is closed, which is against the roof of your mouth with the tip just behind the upper front teeth. It is that simple. And yet, I have noticed that with my tongue in this position my nasal breathing is noticeably better than if my tongue is behind my lower teeth or in any other position. It seems to have some degree of impact on how the airway seals and better handles air through the nose when in this position.

There are a number of other claimed benefits for tongue posture which I cannot really speak to, but for proper breathing and in particular proper breathing during sleep, my experience is that it definitely helps. Give it a try.

Weight Loss

As is discussed in detail elsewhere in this book, excess weight can have a severe negative impact on breathing while asleep by distorting the airway. The tube which makes up our airway is, under normal circumstances, quite rigid and strong resisting being bent, kinked, or flattened. When a person is significantly over weight however, pressure is exerted by the additional weight inwardly against the tube with significant force causing it to become more easily distorted, particularly when the body is in a lying position. Additional weight can also more easily flatten or kink the airway causing obstruction.

The disruption of restful sleep then has the effect of disrupting hormonal regulation of hunger making the sleep deprived person consume more food than necessary while awake and exacerbating the issue. As such, if you are overweight, losing weight may be the number one thing that can improve your sleep. In many instances, people caught in this vicious cycle are able to use CPAP or BIPAP to improve their sleep and then concurrently lose weight until they no longer need the machine to sleep well and maintain the more suitable weight. I have seen cases where the simple use of CPAP allowed a subject to lose over 100 pounds and completely resolve their sleep apnea and constant hunger issues allowing them to resume exercising and achieve/maintain a healthy weight long term. Obesity and sleep loss are tied closely to each other – fixing one greatly helps to fix the other.

Breathing Aides for Sleep - Surgical

If temporary measures give you some degree of relief, but you are still not getting full nasal breathing capacity at all times, you should see a doctor (specifically, an otolaryngologist or Ear, Nose, and Throat specialist, better known as an ENT) to determine if you may be a candidate for any of a number of surgical procedures which may greatly improve your ability to breathe. In the vast majority of cases, these procedures are covered by insurance because health insurance companies are fully aware of the long-term effects of obstructed breathing and impaired sleep. These are just some of the procedures available – there are many others with new ones coming along all the time.

Septoplasty

Septoplasty is the surgical repair/straightening of a deviated septum. The septum is the bony divider in the nose separating the two nasal airways. While it is frequently performed in conjunction with the commonly known rhinoplasty (or "nose job" as it is more commonly known), it is neither the same thing nor done for the same reason.

Generally speaking, rhinoplasty is concerned with the cartilage "tenting" structure of the nose and the draping of skin over it for aesthetics. Unlike most rhinoplasty, septoplasty can be performed without the associated longer healing time, discoloration and swelling to the area of the eyes associated with rhinoplasty. A word of caution to anyone contemplating cosmetic rhinoplasty: you would be well advised to seek a plastic surgeon who is also an ENT or at a minimum who has detailed understanding of breathing issues as related to rhinoplasty. It is not unusual for a patient's breathing to be negatively impacted by a rhinoplasty and, in my experience, this happens far more often in the care of a plastic surgeon than a surgeon who is an ENT or both.

A rhinoplasty alone will not generally improve your nasal breathing at all and, in many cases, can make it far worse. I do, however, know plastic surgeons who make a concerted effort to never degrade and, wherever possible, improve a patient's breathing in conjunction with this cosmetic procedure – do your research carefully.

Turbinate Reduction

Turbinates are the fleshy structures inside the sinus cavities which induce turbulence into the airflow and humidify the incoming air when we breathe. Think of the space inside the nasal passages and sinuses as a maze and the turbinates are the interior walls of that maze. Their purpose is to disrupt the flow of air, moisturize it and cause it to become more turbulent (hence the name) and, in doing so improve, the temperature, water content, and usability of incoming air. In some cases, especially when there is a deviated septum, turbinates can swell to a size which impedes normal airflow. (I had this issue.)

This can be corrected by various methods of reducing the turbinate structures surgically. Some methods are done on an outpatient procedure with electrocautery whereas surgical intervention may be necessary in more advanced cases. Turbinate reduction is often done in conjunction with septoplasty because a deviated septum often results in sympathetic overcompensation of the turbinate structures on the larger side of the septum. They essentially swell to fill in the added space available and must be reduced back to normal when the septum is straightened. Since one side of the nasal cavity is compressed reducing its airflow, when the other side overcompensates by enlarging its turbinates, airflow is significantly reduced on both sides. This is why those with a deviated septum generally have poor airflow on both sides as opposed to good on one side and poor on the other - it negatively impacts both sides.

When either the turbinates, the soft palate/uvula area or the base of the tongue are treated via electrocautery to improve breathing during sleep, this is often referred to as somnoplasty. This is a less invasive method which is often tried first or in less severe cases to correct issues in these areas. I personally had somnoplasty of the turbinates before determining that a more extensive surgical correction would be necessary. Others I know had sufficient improvement from just somnoplasty.

Ethmoidectomy

The ethmoid sinus cavity is a small chamber located at the top rear area of the main sinus and has a small entrance. Ethmoidectomy essentially removes the barrier wall and annexes this additional space as part of the major sinus area, giving a larger sinus space and better airflow. Ethmoidectomy is often performed in conjunction with septoplasty and turbinate reduction. When I had surgery, it included all of these as well as stiffening pillars in the soft palate area.

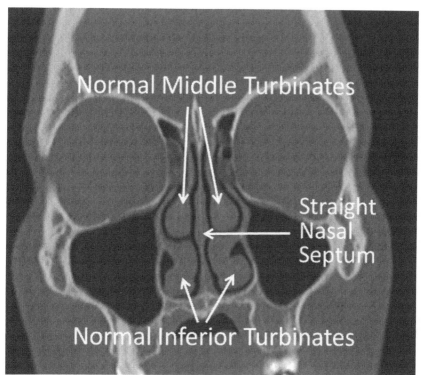

Normal septum and turbinates.

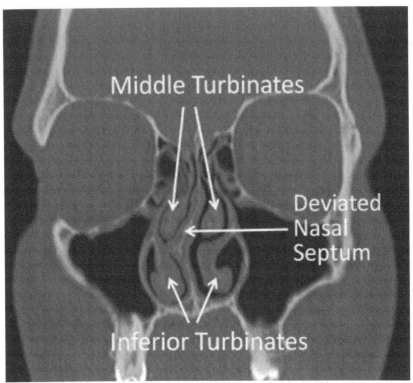

Deviated Septum and compressed/enlarged turbinates.

UPPP

Uvulopalatopharyngoplasty (UPPP) is a procedure that removes excess tissue in the throat to make the airway entrance wider. It involves removal of significant amounts of soft tissue from the throat which may include the uvula, part of the roof of the mouth, and excess throat tissue. I have heard this procedure described as "being carved out like a pumpkin" by more than a few people who have had it and have universally heard that the recovery is *extremely* painful and difficult. To date I have avoided having this procedure but have not ruled out the possibility that I may need it in the future. There is some promise that lasers may prove effective in reducing the invasiveness and recovery time/pain involved in this surgery, but to date this has not come to pass. There are varying degrees of this type of procedure with some involving more tissue removal than others. I was told by some who had it that the first days of the recovery are the most difficult because it is exceedingly painful to swallow which makes it difficult to take pain medications. Several of these patients told me that liquid forms of Vicodin or other pain medications made this considerably easier to do, so bear this in mind if you are ever considering this procedure.

Pillar Procedure (stiffening rods)

A relatively new procedure, this technique is quite simple. It involves a surgeon placing stiff fiberglass or plastic rods into the soft tissue at the back of the throat where they remain permanently. The rods add stiffness to the palate and, as time goes by, scar tissue forms around them increasing stiffness of the tissue. This hardens the tissue of the soft palate making it less susceptible to vibration reducing snoring and airway collapse/obstruction in this area. The procedure is often included as part of a multi-modal surgical approach including turbinate reduction, septoplasty, etc. I personally had this procedure included with my septoplasty and turbinate reduction and in truth couldn't really feel anything from it afterward. It was definitely helpful with really no pain or recovery that I could notice.

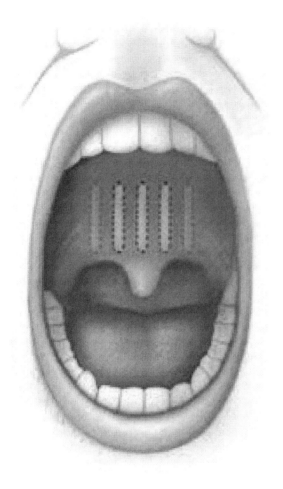

Pillars can be surgically implanted into the tissue of the soft palate to reduce its ability to vibrate and, as such, decrease airway disruption and snoring.

Things I Have Tested Which Consistently Improve Sleep

You will recall that I mentioned that sleep metrics allow us to test different things to see which help us sleep better. To date, I have tested no less than 50 different such things. The way I test them is by defining a sleep note for each sleep aide I try and, whenever I use it, making a note in Sleep Cycle when I go to bed and start the app. Over the past 2000+ nights, I have accumulated a body of data on the sleep aides I have tested. Here are some very consistently effective things I have tested which you can use quite easily. A description of each follows the graph:

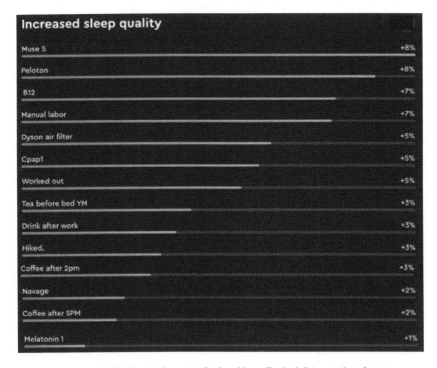

Increased sleep quality	
Muse 5	+8%
Peloton	+8%
B12	+7%
Manual labor	+7%
Dyson air filter	+5%
Cpap1	+5%
Worked out	+5%
Tea before bed YM	+3%
Drink after work	+3%
Hiked.	+3%
Coffee after 2pm	+3%
Navage	+2%
Coffee after 5PM	+2%
Melatonin 1	+1%

My Sleep Cycle notes graphed over time to track what things effectively improve sleep for me.

Before I address each of these, I will mention that this list is only a cross-section of some of the most time-tested and effective sleep interventions I've tested. I have left out several I've either not tested long enough for the data to normalize (with a 2000-night base this takes a while nowadays...), or which are more experimental and not for everyone. One of these I will discuss last of all. Even though it is still too early to ascertain its efficacy, the early results are extremely promising! The items in the chart above have all been verified over multiple years at this point and I consider them solid, reliable performers. There are also potential interaction and cross purpose effects possible, so I have tested many of these things individually and in combinations over time and tried to only ever add one new thing at a time to an established collection of things I am using at a given time. Even so, I have achieved incredible improvement consistently from many of these things and I suspect you will as well, so let's go through some of the best ones now so you can try them yourself.

Muse 5: 8% improvement. This is one of the most astounding things I have ever tested and achieved immediate, good results from. Muse is a specific device and app for practicing Transcendental Meditation and using it only 5 minutes a night before sleep has had this consistent, strong improvement for me after almost 2 years of use. I have been trying to learn and master TM for years, but was never able to make any real progress until I started using the Muse system. It may not be necessary at all for others and it may very well be that simply doing 5 minutes of good meditation will get you the same or better results, but I cannot say. I have trouble even doing 5 minutes – after 2 years I have yet to simply increase it to 10 or even 7, but I plan to over time. Any way you slice it, this 5 minutes of meditation before sleep has yielded a solid and reliable sleep improvement and is consistent over time. I have also recorded a 30-point drop in my blood pressure after doing this same 5-minute practice, which may very well be related to its effect on sleep.

Peloton: +8% improvement.   Once again, this is my specific implementation of something that can be done many ways. Peloton is a stationary exercise bike, but I get similar if not equal or better results riding my road bike for the same time -I am just not able to do it as often. Since I ride the Peloton bike the most, I give it the attribution here. Make no mistake about it: exercise improves sleep. I have broken my exercise into basically 3 different types. I only do one on any given day and all three types improve my sleep significantly. The improvements I achieve through exercise do not require extreme exertion, either. Most of my peloton rides have been 20 minutes these past 2 years and it is only recently that I have started moving up to 30 minutes – once or twice a week. I have come to believe that, long term, optimal sleep cannot be achieved without regular exercise.

B12: +7% This was and still is a surprise discovery. About two years back I glanced at my regular lab blood testing and noticed I had developed a B12 deficiency. I did some research and learned this might be a cause of some minor issues I'd been experiencing, so I began taking supplemental B12 by subcutaneous injection weekly. (another thing I do myself which most of you will want to see a physician for) To my surprise, on the days when I injected B12, my sleep score jumped and has done so consistently. I have not done much research into why this might be the case, but it clearly is, at least for me. This is one of those things that most people will need a doctor's input and assistance for.

Manual Labor: 7% Manual labor is my second exercise classification. I define it as an hour or more doing really exhausting work, such as chopping firewood, digging, construction, and a few other things that I do around my house that make me drench my clothes in sweat and pass out early at bedtime. If you do this kind of thing with any regularity, give yourself credit for exercise on those days and enjoy a good night's sleep.

Dyson Air Filter: 5%   This was another unexpected surprise I stumbled onto. I bought the Dyson air filter/heater a few years back to heat my bedroom on a few really cold days a year and to clean the air every day and night. It has yielded a consistent 5% improvement, and I have seen literature supporting better sleep when air is purified, so it makes sense. This is an easy way to improve your sleep environment. The Dyson is my specific implementation for a room HEPA filter but other air cleaners may work just as well.

CPAP: 5% (Continuous Positive Airway Pressure.) This is something most people may not ever need, but when I resumed snoring it was a life saver. The numbers have normalized since its initial implementation but, back when I first began using this, they were around 18% improvement as it took me from 90 minutes of snoring per night to zero immediately. If I stopped using it before having my throat issue surgically repaired, my snoring would resume and my sleep quality would plummet. I strongly encourage anyone with a snoring issue to test and/or use CPAP until it can be permanently corrected. It's a lifesaver and the nasal only versions (as opposed to full face mask) are much more tolerable and often will do the job. Mouth taping can also be used in conjunction with a nasal only mask.

Worked out: 5%   This is my third form of exercise – resistance training with weights for about an hour in my home gym. Usually I do this 2-3 times a week on a 3-way split schedule so body parts have full time to recover before training again. This number has normalized down a bit but can get as high as 10%. Exercise overall is one of the best sleep aides available, period.

Tea before bed: 3% This is something that I only do about half the year when it is cold enough to be comfortable with a warm drink before sleep. I believe that if I did it every night all year long the score would be much higher. I simply drink one cup of hot Yerba Mate tea with about a tablespoon of honey in it and I really drift off to sleep fast and sleep well. The surprising thing here is that Yerba Mate tea has caffeine in it, yet this works great. I have seen a few studies which concluded that a subject who drinks a caffeinated beverage and then sleeps will consistently get better sleep than one who sleeps and then has a caffeinated beverage upon waking. (This was studied in daytime naps.) It seems that there may be some mechanism by which the caffeine actually assists with entering more restful sleep states by becoming bioavailable after you are already asleep – possibly by making the brain more active during sleep. All I can say is that when I take tea this way, I am sleepy by the end of the cup, quickly fall asleep, and some nights the improvement has been 10%. For me, this works, especially in fall and winter. In summer it isn't something I can do as I cannot sleep when I am too warm, so I forego this from about March to October unless there's an unusually cold night.

Hiking: 3% I alternate hiking 1 mile (half uphill, half downhill) with my other cardio but only in the cooler fall and winter months, so it averages out lower than it really is when I do it. Hiking was one of the first forms of exercise that I noticed improved my sleep. It is a nice combination for cardio and strength depending on the terrain and can improve my sleep 8% or more.

Drink after work: 3% This is another surprise discovery that is consistent. On days when I have one (just one) drink (a beer or one mixed cocktail) either after work or with dinner, I sleep 3% or more better. What can I say, alcohol in moderation would appear to aide sleep.

Coffee After 2PM: 3% Another surprising and consistent result. A lot of what we have been told about caffeinated drinks is just wrong. When I drink coffee after 2PM but no later than 5PM, I sleep better. I believe there is a reason for this; when I am tiring out early in the day, I could rest or I can try to push through. It is my belief that using caffeine and pushing through consolidates my waking hours somewhat so that, when I do finally get to sleep, my "tired time" has been consolidated to my sleep hours. Similarly, I have learned that when I am tired near bedtime to NOT push through and keep doing things because that will lead to my becoming awake and then having trouble sleeping. If we simply keep ourselves awake during daylight and sleep at night, things work better and caffeine in the late afternoon can assist with this quite effectively.

I have begun to believe that the window where coffee or other caffeinated drinks will negatively affect sleep is in the 2-3 hours before going to bed. Before this, caffeine seems to actually help sleep (via waking hour consolidation as I previously mentioned) and immediately before bed has the positive effect I have described with Yerba Mate Tea. These dynamics should become clearer from my data over time and, again, there will be some variation among individuals, but I think this is generally what is correct. My research continues…

Navage: 2% Navage is the powered nasal rinse system I discuss in the breathing aides section. I went a year or more without using it and then resumed so its true number is certainly higher – probably around 5-6%. (I forgot to clean it and it became slightly moldy and had to be completely sanitized – ALWAYS break down and clean the unit after use and before storage!) There is no question that I breathe and sleep better every time that I use this. And it leaves me feeling really good for going to sleep – the fresh scent and feeling of the rinse has become a kind of ritual for heading to bed and sleeping well.

Melatonin: 1% This refers to a single 300mcg dose tablet of melatonin at bed time. I have always liked the Sundown brand. Melatonin is the hormone we naturally produce when blue light stops hitting our retinas after sunset – it tells us to start moving towards sleep. This metric is a bit deceptive because melatonin really shines in helping me to fall asleep as opposed to sleep quality, which is what this hormone is supposed to do. There is no question that I fall asleep faster when I take this, and when I forget I often notice. Within about 20 minutes, I just find it easy to drift off to sleep. If for any reason I should need to though, I can stay awake through it just by trying. It is a small thing, but that ease of getting to sleep makes melatonin a real win in my book.

Tetris: 8-9% This is one of the newest things I have been testing so it does not appear in my graphs as yet, but I include it here because it shows great promise. Over the last decade, multiple neuroscience researchers have found beneficial links between playing the video game Tetris and certain cognitive functions. After hearing that there were applications of using the game for as little as 5 minutes to improve relaxation, I began testing it at bedtime. While I have only accumulated some 30 days of test data at the time of this writing, my five-minute nightly tests using Tetris have uniformly improved sleep quality by 8-9% every time. While this needs more testing before I can conclusively recommend it, Tetris for 5 minutes is the most promising new sleep aide I have tested in quite a while! It's free, and has no downside I am aware of, so give it a try.

The Night Environment and Falling Asleep

Falling asleep each night is the first half of the equation in a good night's sleep, the other half is staying asleep. These are generally the two things we all have difficulty with. Like so many things which animals in the wild and most of our domesticated pets still know how to do properly by instinct, falling asleep is yet another natural process that we have un-learned how to do over the past 100+ years.

The first thing we need to learn about how to fall asleep properly ties directly into how to wake up properly, and it involves the presence of external stimuli: light and sound.

Our ongoing erosion of proper sleep patterns and procedures has led us to a point where we often need to use loud, harsh audible alarms to arouse us from sleep in the morning. Everything about this practice is wrong. I have not used an alarm, other than for an unusual and unavoidable event (like having to leave home at 5AM to catch a plane) in about 10 years. Today I simply won't take a flight that early – sleeping well is more important to me, period. I stopped using an alarm to wake before I began my research into better sleep when I heard something that made immediate sense to me at a time when I was first becoming aware of my need for better sleep. It was simple: somewhere I heard a sleep specialist say that if you need to use an alarm to wake up, you aren't getting enough sleep. That was all I needed to hear – I immediately knew it was true. In the wild, animals like dogs, wolves, bears, etc. don't need alarm clocks – they wake with the morning sun when they've had enough rest as they've done for millions of years. They haven't developed electric lights and sophisticated shelters to deprive themselves of knowing what time of day or night it actually is to their detriment. As such, animals go to sleep at the same relative time EVERY single night of their lives and get a sufficient night's rest to wake up naturally, well rested, when the sun comes up. We need to learn to do the same.

For this reason, I got rid of my morning alarm permanently and started doing effectively the opposite: setting an evening alarm to remind me to get to bed by 11PM. This evolved after my early Sleep Cycle charts revealed that the earlier and more consistently I got to bed before 11PM, the better I slept. This habit is one I have continued to this day. I wake up naturally every day and I use an alarm to remind me when to go to sleep instead of when to wake up. This has become a very simple thing to do with today's smartphones. After having spent time researching my sleep metrics and determining how much time I need to sleep every night, which is about 7.5 - 8 hours, I determined a 1-hour range during which I need to get to bed each night, which for me is 10:30 – 11:30. This allows me to wake up, generally, somewhere around 7:30 AM which is a very good average time for me whatever time of year (and daylight time adjustment) it may currently be. Note: there is margin for variance in both the time I actually get to sleep and the time I wake up. I might get to sleep by 10:30 and might not wake up until 8:30, but generally 11:30 to 7:30 is when I sleep. We all need some margin for error here and you want to build some in to your routine. I always, however, want there to be light outside hen I wake up as I believe there is a negative natural effect to waking up while the sun is still down. Try to obey circadian cycle at all times.

Light

Controlling light as the day winds from sundown to bedtime is a crucial necessity that I learned to master over 5+ years. Only looking back can I now clearly see how important it was and how much it contributes to my ability to sleep well every night.

The spectrum of light visible to humans runs from primarily blue at one end to primarily red at the other. These light color frequencies are the anchors of the two ends of the circadian cycle: night and day or sleep and wake. During the day, we are awakened by and bathed in primarily blue, bright light. This wavelength of light hits specific receptors in our retina from the very first rays we awaken to and tells our physiological systems to become and stay alert. Your eyes need not even be open when this happens – lab research has verified that the body itself can detect and is affected by the bluer wavelengths of light striking it. As previously mentioned, every cell in the body is aware of circadian cycle, which supports this finding.

Many people today are aware of the need for a room as dark as possible all night to facilitate sleep, but that is only half the battle in management of light for proper sleep. Once the sun goes down, we need to gradually eliminate all blue light sources around us to the best of our ability until we go to sleep. 7 years ago, this was hard to do - today it is easy. I first realized this would be useful about 6 years ago. My first focus was on my computer and device screens and long before Night Shift and similar features were built into IOS and other operating systems an excellent program called f.lux came to my attention and I began using it on all my devices. (justgetflux.com) f.lux gradually removes the bluer wavelengths of light from your device's display as the sun goes down in concert with the day's sunset schedule in whatever region of the world you are in, thus keeping your circadian rhythms in tune with the natural cycle of sunlight. This is an excellent tool and I believe that it should be applied to all screens and light sources we use and hope it one day evolves into that – we are getting there gradually. I could easily imagine a home where all the lighting, phones, clocks, screens and devices were graduated in this way in unison to keep our natural sleep patterns working. Actually, I live in such a home. The outdoor sunset each day is followed by a coordinated indoor dimming and blue light removal of ALL my lighted devices every day.

After my first experience using f.lux to dim my screens, at some point I moved to using Phillips HUE light bulbs in my home. These bulbs have WiFi control capability and can be dimmed and/or have their color set remotely. f.lux has the ingenius capability to control these lights automatically so, as the sun sets, every device screen and light in my home start gradually shifting to dimmer and redder frequencies of light. Under master control of f.lux, eventually an hour or two after sunset all lighted devices are devoid of blue light and dimed significantly. Before f.lux and HUE I would do this manually by dimming screens and shifting color on TVs and dimming my lights manually, and I still do that when away from home.

After more than six years of keeping my lighting properly controlled in this manner, I have noticed that my eyes have come *to expect* this to happen after sunset. If I am working at an undimmed computer screen an hour or two after sunset, my eyes start to feel a burning strain reminding me to adjust the lighting. I believe I have reprogrammed the visual portion of my circadian cycle to some degree, and it feels very natural.

Manufacturers are already working to include this technology in television sets and monitors and I predict that it will be a standard feature within 5 years. There are also devices available which TV inputs (like HDMI) can be run through to achieve this same effect with the push of a remote button. If you are like me, you can feel the jarring effect of the blue light from an undimmed tv in your dark bedroom. Dim it and adjust the color as much as needed to make it about the brightness and color of a small campfire and you will have little trouble dozing off to it.

Sound

Sound is the other environmental variable we must control in order to get good sleep every night. This one is a bit easier to control than light, thankfully.

It is easy to believe that a quieter environment is the simplest way to control sound for getting to sleep, but in my experience, wherever you go there can always be something to interfere with what would otherwise be a quiet environment. Human beings, sadly, are a damned noisy species, and as population increases it is getting harder and harder to find quiet places, not only for us but for all other species as well. Recent studies have determined that even marine animals are becoming hyper stressed due to all the noise we are putting into the oceans. Until population increase backs off, noise on this planet will likely keep getting worse.

Fortunately, the human physique is a lot better about shutting out noise while asleep than light. It is mostly during the time we are falling asleep that noise can be most disruptive – once we are asleep, we can sleep through a surprisingly wide variety of loud noise. This is likely an evolved trait – the savannah is full of noises at night.

I am particularly noise sensitive and always have been. As such, I use two things to help me get to sleep easily. The first is that I watch TV on a timer. I will get into details about that ahead because I know most people have heard a lot of incorrect recommendations about television and sleep. On any night when this simple bit of background noise isn't sufficient for me to get to sleep, (which is many) I use industrial foam earplugs, such as those made by 3M. Properly used, these literally seal out all noise. I find I can put in just one and then selectively roll my open ear more or less onto the pillow to be able to hear the tv more or block out all sound. As I lose interest in the TV, I tend to roll onto that open ear and hear nothing and then I'm off to sleep. Properly used (you have to roll them tightly and insert them well into the ear canal where they expand and seal out sound), these earplugs work like magic. There exist a variety of hard to soft such earplugs. You may need to experiment with different softness grades of them to get a good seal and not hurt the bony structure of your ears after several hours.

Temperature

Temperature is a crucial factor in proper sleep. Something I noticed a long time ago is counterintuitive for many people, which is the fact that you can sleep practically no matter how cold it is but not if it is too warm. In my lifetime, I have awakened many times when I was too hot or not been able to fall asleep because it was too hot, but never have I awakened or been unable to fall asleep because I was too cold. Indeed, a basic element of cold weather survival training is that you MUST not fall asleep when exposed to extreme cold because you may never wake up and cold makes us want to sleep. When people die of exposure, this is the last thing they do – fall asleep. The path to the top of Mount Everest is littered with over 200 frozen dead climbers. Many of them are sitting or lying in what look like perfectly natural resting positions, because they are. They stopped to rest, gave in to sleep, and remain there forever because they cannot be retrieved. Sleep thrives in cold and is thwarted by heat.

A large part of this is undoubtedly because body temperature naturally decreases during sleep. While the reasons for this are not entirely understood, it is unquestionably because the biological processes which take place while we are asleep require it. As such, the cooler you can stay while asleep, the better you will generally sleep. Studies have suggested 60 degrees, seemingly quite cold to many people, as an ideal room temperature. I have also read studies showing that the less clothing one wears while asleep, the better the body can radiate heat and the better you will sleep. I have done sleep tracking tests and found this to be true. However, I mostly am only comfortable doing this in the hottest part of summer, so I have little data on it – I generally feel more comfortable with more covering for some reason.

There are numerous different strategies for keeping cool while sleeping in the warmer months. I have found that a ceiling fan above my bed is extremely helpful as is the ability to control my air conditioning from a bedside remote if needed. A bed cooling device called the Chili Pad has received high ratings from some users, but I have not tested it. Its principal seems very sound.

Generally speaking, the thing to remember is to err on the side of cold for better sleep. You will wake up if you get too warm, but not if you are too cold because there really is no such thing unless you are out in the snow somewhere...

Falling Asleep To TV

One need look no further than late night television to see one of the most obvious battlefields in the war on sleep. As recently as the late 1970s, late night television was something that ended at about 1AM and didn't resume until around 7AM the next morning. You heard me right – there was NO tv to watch at night anywhere. Anyone old enough remembers well that if you watched tv late enough back then, at 1AM you'd see something along the lines of an American flag waving in the breeze while some patriotic words were read, the national anthem was played, or a fighter jet blasting through clouds in the blue sky while the words of the poem "High Flight" were read. Then, a test tone would sound while a test pattern filled the screen and this would give way to a screen of "snow" and speaker full of static until early the next morning. (maybe 6 or 7 AM) In case you are too young to have ever seen this, Google search "late night tv signoffs" for a look at this bygone era.

I vaguely remember the beginning of the end of this era. It came about in around 1979 when American citizens living and working in Tehran, Iran, were taken hostage by Islamic extremists. ABC news began holding a nightly news coverage of this ongoing event – an extension of their late national news program - called "America Held Hostage: Day n" where the day number n would go up by one every day. After over a year of this captivity coverage, hosted by news anchor Ted Koppel, the hostages were released very shortly after Ronald Reagan was elected president in 1980. It would have been natural for the special coverage to end, but ABC News had discovered a market for people interested in watching news after hours and the program known as ABC News Nightline was born.

By the time Ted Koppel retired as Nightline's anchor 25 years later in 2005, not only were network sign offs a thing of the past, but we had gone from 4 or 5 broadcast channels which shut down overnight to hundreds of channels, including numerous all-news channels, which remained on the air 24 hours a day, every day. A huge battle in the War on Sleep had been lost and we now live in a society that never knows a blank screen full of static. 24 hours a day, 365 days a year, hundreds of TV channels are a click away. And not just at home anymore – they are with us pretty much anyplace we are.

There has been a lot of discussion over the years about whether or not falling asleep to television is a good or bad idea. Most of what I have seen would argue for it being bad. I personally do not feel that there is anything wrong with falling asleep to TV so long as you do it under certain conditions that make it much more effective while eliminating the potential negatives. I have been falling asleep to tv for many years and I believe I have taken doing so to a point where it is highly effective for me with no downside. Indeed, during just about all of my 2000 nights of recorded sleep analysis, I fell asleep by watching TV, including the present-day scores which average above 90%.

The first argument against tv as sleep aide is that the light from the screen being emitted into your eyes is not sleep conducive, which is true. In fact, the specific argument is that the bluer shades of light have the same effect as daytime sunlight which is that these wavelengths of light trigger the portion of our circadian cycle that says, "wake up, be alert, time to work." However, let's look at this in context. If we want to emulate a proper daily circadian rhythm the way animals still do, and the way our ancestors did, the idea is to have a gradually decreasing level of light (and sound) that ultimately gives way to total darkness (and near silence, though it's never completely quiet out in the wilderness) as we fall asleep at the end of the day. As such, I go from a fully lit house to a bedroom lit only by the (dimmed) light of a tv screen with the blue spectrum eliminated as I drift off to sleep. This is not, incidentally, unlike how our ancestors ended the day heading to sleep by a fire – a source of mostly red light and subtle sounds in one spot nearby their sleeping spot. In order to do this effectively, I adhere to some specific things which I have evolved over the past decade:

1) The tv screen is dimmed (via the brightness, backlight, color and contrast settings) to as low as I can get it and still see the screen. This cuts greatly the amount of light hitting my retinas and working to keep me awake. Newer televisions often have preset configurations so I have one I call "sleep" which has these parameters preset. The goal is to remove as much of the bluer wavelengths of light as possible and this has been a very effective way to do that for me. There are also special glasses available which filter all light reaching the eyes to remove the type of light that stimulates you to stay awake. (again, the bluer wavelengths) These are known as blue light blocking glasses, and they ostensibly filter out the blue spectra of light which prevent you from easily sleeping. I have found these glasses, however, to be mostly ineffective. Because they only block light coming from straight ahead, blue and bright light can and does still get to your eyes from the sides. As such, my recommendation is that if you are in a place where you cannot control the sources of light (a Hotel, friend's house, etc.) then such glasses are better than nothing, but controlling the light sources will always be the better option by a wide margin.

2) I watch only specific kinds of shows or movies and only from pre-recorded sources. This is because I want to keep the sound levels low and consistent. All it takes is one blasting commercial during an otherwise quiet program to jolt you right out of a good sleep state and ruin your entire night's sleep. I have learned that certain types of shows are far more conducive to relaxation and falling asleep than others, and I watch those shows and only from sources (Netflix, downloads, etc.) with no commercial interruptions. While you will find whatever works for you, I avoid action shows, any reality tv, things involving music, news, anything with too much action and chaos. I find that old tv series and movies (from the 70s and earlier) tend to be more conducive to this purpose. They were made in a pre-MTV era when the audience didn't have to be constantly jarred to keep paying attention. Mysteries and crime dramas really just put me out – Columbo (Seasons 1-7) is a favorite I have fallen asleep to literally hundreds of times! You will find what works best for you by experimenting. Also, as I mention elsewhere, we are programmed to fall asleep faster by a fire so videos of fires burning are readily available and will definitely help you fall asleep.

3) Volume levels need to be kept low and, if possible, set to limit any volume spikes. Some newer TVs have controls for this which are great.

4) Headphones or earphones are fine and for me are especially useful when I do not have a quiet environment. When I travel, my laptop computer on the bed with earbuds works great. If having something on or in your ears bothers you during sleep, look into a pillow speaker.

5) A sleep timer to shut off the TV is a must. If it is running all night it WILL wake you up and ruin your sleep cycle at some point. Many nights, I find myself drifting off and just hit the power button but I always have the timer set for 90 minutes.

6) It is better, if possible, to watch in a position in which you would naturally lay while falling asleep. Remember, your view doesn't have to be perfect – you're going to start closing your eyes and just listening at some point. I usually pick up the show the next night from wherever I passed out the night before, and it works great for me. I should note that every time I have had a perfect 100% sleep score, I fell asleep watching TV in this manner. Most if not all of my 2000 recorded nights I fell asleep this way.

In over a decade of using TV to fall asleep, these are the tips I have developed. I find that it is a very good way to transition from the busy day where I need to be highly alert to the quiet evening where I want to slip off into sleep. If you, like me, can follow these guidelines and use TV to fall asleep quickly and easily, then by all means do so. It has been a wonderful sleep aide for me for a long time.

Audio Books

Listening to audio books is another method of falling asleep that I have found to work very well. The "bedtime story" is a long-known method of becoming relaxed and lulled to sleep that we all know of going back to childhood. (when we used to sleep much better!) For me this tends to work even better when I need to nap during the day, when tv would not.

Eating Before Sleep

It's one of those things I hear people, especially those more conscious of their weight and subject to every untested fad, parroting over and over again: don't eat within a few hours of bedtime. The exact number of hours and the reasons vary. I usually hear from one to five hours and either because it will cause you to gain weight or because it will interfere with your sleep. Both are generally complete nonsense.

Let's start with the one I have heard more often which is that eating before bedtime will cause you to gain weight. What, exactly, is this based on? There is ZERO scientific evidence of this that I am aware of. Your bodyweight and/or bodyfat as a percent of body composition are based on a very simple set of factors: How much and what type of food you ingest, how much exercise you get, genetics and, as we are learning, how well you sleep. If you eat 2000 calories per day and don't vary your exercise or sleep, it makes absolutely *no discernable difference* what time during your waking hours you ingest those calories. None. Primitive man, until sometime before the War on Sleep began, ate whenever it was convenient – when food could be found, when a kill was made, or when another had food to share. Our ancestors didn't worry about how fat they were getting and, in fact, they were better off if they were carrying some fat because intermittent fasting was inevitable when food became scarce. There is scant if any evidence of obesity in our distant predecessors. You can be certain that a day spent tracking and killing game frequently ended with a large meal cooked over an open fire after which they fell asleep. They ate when they were hungry, in varying amounts, and at whatever time they cared to or could, and that is what we should do as well. I have seen documentaries shot in the 1980s about the Waorani indigenous people of the Ecuadorian rainforest who still live much as they did thousands of years ago. In one segment, they spent most of a day hunting and pursuing a howler monkey across 20+ miles of terrain before killing it, climbing 50+ feet into the canopy to claim it, and returning home. I promise you; they ate heartily before bed that night. (See the excellent 1984 PBS documentary "Nomads of the Rain Forest" to learn more and see how we lived not long ago.)

As for eating interfering with sleep, all evidence contradicts this when there are not digestive issues (such as GERD which was previously mentioned) involved. Consider: how many times have you left work for lunch, only to fight to stay awake for the rest of the afternoon when you got back? The digestion of food is an energy consuming process. To digest food you have eaten, your body has to divert energy from other things, which is why it is natural to feel sleepy after a meal, especially the later in the day it is consumed. When we eat breakfast, we've been asleep and not eating for 8 or more hours, so the effect is mostly opposite at this time of day. The often-heard tome of breakfast being the most important meal of the day is quite likely correct. Since your stores are depleted after waking, a good breakfast will bring up your energy levels rather than deplete them. If you watch any of the television reality shows where people engage in survival scenarios, such as Man vs. Wild, Survivorman, or Naked and Afraid, you will frequently hear participants who have been starving for days remark after finally eating how they "feel the energy flowing back into their body". (In these shows, particularly Naked and Afraid, participants rapidly fall into a lifestyle strikingly similar to the aforementioned Waorani people and give us a very useful look into how we are meant to live, eat and sleep naturally.) I have done some survival training and experienced this. As our day wears on and we engage in activity, lunch has somewhat of a tradeoff of energy gained vs. lost which is why, in many cultures around the world, a siesta after lunch is customary. If you've ever taken a post lunch siesta, you were probably amazed at how much better your energy level was afterward for the rest of the day. I try to keep lunch on the light side so as to avoid this dynamic unless I expect to engage in heavy manual labor or exercise after lunch.

By the time dinnertime rolls around, we are generally ready for the largest meal of our day after having done the bulk of our mental and physical exertion for the day. Incidentally, while it comprises only around 2% of our body mass, the brain uses more than 20% of the calories we ingest. (!) When you sit and do mentally taxing work and notice you are becoming hungry after some time, that is no coincidence: thinking burns calories – this has been measured in laboratory research.   After this final meal of the day, it is very probable that we will be feeling sleepy within a few hours.   The reasons are obvious: we've been exerting ourselves all day and now it's time for our body to spend all night recovering, repairing, and digesting, which will consume so much energy we won't even be conscious. Circadian cycle even shuts off our need to move our bowels at night – a clear indicator that we are likely meant to eat up until bedtime and digest during sleep. Not only is eating before bed not a bad idea, I believe it's a very logical idea and what nature most likely intended us to do. Many times, I've awoken from sleep in the middle of the night or could not fall asleep when I was hungry, but I have never awoken because I was too full. Quite the contrary. Do as our ancestors did: eat when you are hungry and let nature take care of the rest. Don't listen to the unfounded, clichéd advice parroted by people with no practical knowledge or evidence.

Wakefulness Aides

In the same way that substances like melatonin are extremely useful for helping your body learn to sleep at the right time, wakefulness aides can be utilized in a prudent and reasonable manner to assist in adjusting your body to maximum alertness during proper waking hours. Prolonged or frequent use of some wakefulness aides or combinations of aides however can be a sign that other problems exist, so your use of them should be tracked and moderated. There are some days when no matter how well I have slept I cannot get myself to optimum performance without something to improve my alertness and focus. Other days the thought never even crosses my mind. For our intents and purposes, wakefulness aides, like sleep aides, serve a very valid function. Here are some of the ones which I use on some regular basis.

Bulletproof Coffee

Bulletproof coffee is both a generic term and a brand description for a specific way of making coffee blended with grass-fed butter and MCT (Medium Chain Triglyceride – usually coconut) oil. It has been around for many years, but was first popularized in the mainstream by noted biohacker Dave Asprey a few years ago.

As the story goes, a man was hiking at altitudes around 18,000 feet in Tibet and was near exhaustion when a Sherpa gave him tea that was mixed with yak butter. The tea rejuvenated him so profoundly that he spent years researching it and the result was Bulletproof coffee. You can find the recipe online along with many ways to make it. Basically, it is made by brewing coffee and then adding the butter and MCT oil. Blending this mix in a blender is crucial as it causes a much better mixing of the elements and is much more drinkable. The concoction delivers needed fats in a manner that can stave off hunger and keep you alert and focused for several hours, making it an acceptable meal replacement for many people. I have NEVER in my life been able to skip or shrink my breakfast food requirement but, when drinking Bulletproof coffee, I can do so with no negative impact and go for several hours before needing to eat. As wakefulness aides go, this is one of the best to come along in a very long time.

Modafinil

Modafinil (trade names include Provigil, Modapro, and Modalert) is an extremely interesting drug that has been available for some 30+ years but only become popular as a treatment for sleep related issues in the past 20 years or so. The paradox with the vast majority of stimulants used to offset EDS or narcolepsy (and stimulants in general, for that matter) is that most have significant side effects which must be endured in exchange for their benefits. Generally speaking, the vast majority of stimulants cause a refractory period (or "crash") after their use, they prevent rest or sleep during or for some time after their effective period, or they cause agitation, hunger, and difficulty regulating body temperature. For this reason, using any of them on a regular basis does far more damage than good and even when used properly their benefit is limited.

Modafinil is a nearly complete departure from these classes of drugs. Originally designed for treatment of narcolepsy / EDS (Excessive Daytime Somnolence) it is, for the most part, devoid of the aforementioned side effects. I originally became aware of the drug when I was training as a private pilot and learned from military pilots that it had entirely replaced older amphetamines that had been used by US military aviators since WWII. The astonishing thing about Modafinil is that there are recorded trials where subjects have used it to stay awake 48 or more hours with only a 1-2% loss in performance of complex tasks. What's more, Modafinil has proven to be a "smart drug" which significantly improves focus and mental clarity in most users. For those with EDS, it is pretty much a miracle drug. While I do not recommend it for long term use, it can be extremely effective in helping to adjust rough spots in one's waking hours schedule. Adjusting to an earlier wake time, for example, or offsetting jet lag. Performance improvement during times requiring solid focus and performance (test taking, for example) are well documented and have led to significant abuse of the drug by persons without sleep disorders, much in the same way that Adderall has come to be abused.

While Modafinil is not a long-term solution to sleep issues, it is unquestionably one of the sharper tools in the toolbox of someone who suffers from the debilitating effects of excessive fatigue during the day. Used in conjunction with the techniques described in this book to improve sleep, it can result in a significant improvement in both sleep quality score and productivity/wakefulness/energy levels during awake hours. Before 7 years ago when I first began using metrics and achieved my biggest improvements, I kept Modafinil in supply and used it at least a few times a week. Now, I couldn't tell you the last time I used it. It is a useful tool but, if you follow the advice I present, you will likely never need it. Modafinil is a prescription medication, so obtain and use it only under the supervision of a physician.

(Note: I do not discuss Adderall nor Ritalin in this work because I have never used either and do not intend to. They are not, to my knowledge, prescribed for sleep disorders as Modafinil is and, as such, don't really have any place in a book about sleep that I am aware of.)

Aides for Falling Asleep

Over the past decade, I have had the opportunity to test a great many sleep aides. Over the past six years, I have been able to very closely monitor the effectiveness of these aides, both individually and in concert, by using sleep metrics. The following are my findings based on my ongoing trials of these different things.

Melatonin

Melatonin is a naturally occurring hormone which helps to regulate our circadian rhythm. It is found in animals, plants, fungi, and bacteria. It is widely believed that all living things on Earth are governed by circadian cycles all the way down to the level of individual cells. Melatonin may be the primary chemical that tells our cells, individually and in concert, when it is time to sleep and to wake. Its importance is not to be underestimated.

Because we have greatly disrupted our natural circadian cycle with artificial light and other disruptions, we generally produce and release melatonin into our bloodstream in unnatural amounts and not necessarily at the right times. Everyone has probably heard the story of how if a person goes out into an unmechanized environment, such as camping deep in the woods away from all human contact, their proper, normal circadian cycle becomes restored in about 10 days. This is quite true, and part of what happens in these cases is that the natural production and schedule of melatonin in the body return to normal, proper levels and cycles. We can't all go camping every night to improve our sleep. We can, however, utilize supplemental melatonin to assist us in restoring proper circadian cycles.

I have been using melatonin nightly for most of 7 years now with great results and no side effects. Many people take it expecting it to work like some strong prescription sleeping pill, which is not a realistic expectation. My experience is that 300mcg of melatonin taken just before I want to fall asleep will allow me to fall asleep within about 20-30 minutes easily. It's not a knockout drug – one could easily stay awake after taking it and, in an hour or so in my experience, any effect of helping you to sleep will have passed. As such, I only take it once I'm actually in bed with the lights dimmed preparing to fall asleep.

In over 1000 nights of testing, I receive an average 3% sleep quality improvement from melatonin. Because melatonin is used to get to sleep, I believe its beneficial effect is slightly lost in the tracking statistics. However, make no mistake about it, melatonin helps one to fall asleep quickly and regularly and, taken as properly intended, improves overall circadian cycle and sleep quality. No question about it.

Melatonin also has, in my experience, no detrimental effects and does not impact waking up nor alertness after waking up. I have heard reports of people who had difficulty waking or felt sluggish after using it. In all the cases of this type that I know of, the user exceeded the recommended dosage by many times, which is not a good idea and will not yield good results, and/or did not have enough collected data to draw proper conclusions. After 2000 nights, I believe my conclusions on melatonin are fairly sound.

4-7-8 Breathing

I have to admit that when I first heard about this sleep-inducing technique, I was skeptical. However, since it was simple to do and free to test, I gave it a try immediately and was extremely surprised. This technique definitely works and not only for falling asleep but it is also generally effective for reducing anxiety and can be used anytime, anywhere. In some medical articles I have read that it can be as effective as a dose of Valium in helping a subject to relax and fall asleep – THAT got my attention.

It works like this: you breath in for a count of 4 (it doesn't matter if each count is one second or two or whatever, what matters is that you use the same interval for each count. I use one second generally.), hold that breath for a count of 7, then exhale steadily for a count of 8. Then repeat until you are either calmed down or asleep. Try it now and see how it works.

While I cannot explain exactly how or why this works, I have some idea after doing some experimentation based on the work of Wim Hof, aka 'The Iceman". Without going too far afield, Hof is a master and world record holder in many feats that are seemingly impossible, most all of which involve breathing and extreme cold. He is able to do unbelievable (and verified) things like climbing some of the world's highest peaks in a pair of shorts or staying under the surface of frozen bodies of water and swimming farther than anyone else. He performs these feats by manipulating his breathing to create oxygen deficiency or oversupply in various situations which allow him to perform these seemingly superhuman feats. I believe that the 4-7-8 breathing technique creates a degree of oxygen deficit which tends to calm the body and make one slightly sleepy. It's amazing, it's free, and, in my experience, it works. Give it a try.

How I Sleep Every Night Now

When I first began talking to people in various places – on social media, in special interest groups online, in person, anywhere, two things always seemed to happen: First, it would quickly become apparent that they had significant interest in improving their sleep – I rarely met anyone who said they slept great and had no need for improvement. (and in the rare instances when I did, I usually determined they were actually not but in fact had just convinced themselves they were.)   Secondly, after hearing all I'd accomplished, they wanted to know how I did it.

As tempting as it often was to try to tell them how to do what I had, I quickly realized that trying to help them to do so outside of the context of telling them everything I'd learned and HOW I'd learned it would more than likely not be a good idea. At best, they'd randomly retain a few things that they might try, might not try them correctly, probably wouldn't quantify them, and might even get hurt by them. This quickly made me realize that I needed to write a book to explain all that I had learned in sequence and context so that others could gain the knowledge I had and put it into practice properly and safely.

Now that you have read this book and acquired all that knowledge, I will now tell you what my nightly sleep routine looks like. Currently, my average sleep score in Sleep Cycle across days, weeks, and months is 93%. (remember, in my earliest nights, scores were in the 50s and 60s) At one point during the COVID-19 pandemic, I logged seven nights in a row at 100%, which is a record for me. As I mentioned, I made sleep a focus when the pandemic started and it paid off very quickly and has been sustained. As you've seen, over time I have been gradually and consistently improving my sleep quality, testing different things and tracking their effect using the Sleep Notes feature of Sleep Cycle. I believe that anyone can do this and that tracking and consistency are the main factors once breathing is properly established and any snoring eliminated.

So, without further delay, here is how I get to sleep most every night:

As you know by now, I do not believe in nor use an alarm to wake up in the morning. I set Sleep Cycle to wake me within my desired range, but I almost always (I'd say 8 of 10 mornings) wake up before it does on my own. Instead, I set an alarm on my phone to remind me to go to sleep. That alarm goes off at 10PM each night and my goal is to be in bed within an hour of it going off and to get 8 to 8.5 hours in bed. I came to find long ago that an alarm reminding me to get to bed is FAR more valuable than an alarm trying to jolt me out of REM sleep the next morning. In my opinion, alarm clocks should be banished for waking up and we should all use sleep reminder alarms instead.

My nightly routine actually begins hours before that 11PM alarm goes off, however, having been shaped by years of research and tracking results. If in the afternoon I start running out of gas, I will have coffee (usually the Bulletproof style). This is also true in the early evening – if I am tired and it's too early to sleep and/or I still need to get things done, I will have coffee up until as late as 6 PM. My testing discovered long ago, as you saw in my charts of results, that coffee after 2PM actually consistently improves my sleep quality.

Starting in the hour after sundown, all my phone, computer, lights, and TV screens start to automatically dim under control of f.lux. I am very aware of avoiding any bright lights once this starts and it has become an ingrained habit. This effectively makes my entire house dim in unison as the sun goes down and I transition into bedtime over the hours from Sunset until around 10PM.

In the hour or 2 before bed, I go through a routine of things many people do like brushing my teeth, washing up, and removing my contact lenses. After that, I perform a nasal rinse using the Navage device with warm saline.

I head to bed with my blackout curtains closed and my bedroom lights dimmed to the lowest point of the day. Sitting up in bed, I do my 5 minutes or so of Tetris (currently testing) and then my 5 minutes of transcendental meditation with the Muse headset. Then I take my melatonin tablet.

Next, I set my phone to airplane mode and set it in a charger. I switch my tablet to airplane mode and launch sleep cycle, select my sleep notes for sleep aides, exercise, etc., and start it running and place the tablet on the bedside table.

Lastly, I usually watch blue light free, dimmed tv on timer until I fall asleep. Many nights I'll use one or both earplugs to block out any outdoor noise.

In the rare instance where I have trouble falling asleep at this point, I will practice the 4-7-8 breathing technique. I don't think I've ever done it more than 10 times without going unconscious.

From there, I will usually sleep until I wake up or Sleep Cycle wakes me up. Once in a while I'll wake up thirsty during the night – there's always a bottle of water on my bedside table so I'll drink and go right back to sleep. Occasionally I also might wake up and need to urinate and I'll do so and just go right back to sleep. I don't turn on lights when these things happen and get back to sleep as quickly as possible. I resist all urges to check phones or email or anything – sleep is more important to me and seconds spent awake jeopardize the chance of getting right back to sleep. If I wake up in the am after first light but well before waking time, I will put on a sleep mask to keep myself in darkness and make it easier to fall back to sleep. If I need to use the restroom during this early awakening, I can actually get there and back with the sleep mask on to keep myself in darkness. This makes a huge difference in getting back to sleep.

In the morning, somewhere between 7 and 8, I either wake up on my own or Sleep Cycle gently wakes me while I'm in my shallowest sleep. I never feel lethargic or exhausted – I most always feel really good. If it's a cold time of year, my heat came on around 7 so as to help me wake up after being off to help me sleep. If it's a warm time of year, the AC was on all night to make sure I stayed cool enough to sleep optimally.

Now I turn on my phone, grab my glasses, let in some sunlight to reinforce waking up, and see what happened overnight. By the time that's done, I'm a bit more awake. I grab my water and head to the bathroom where I rinse my mouth out thoroughly and usually use mouthwash or brush my teeth to reduce bacteria that accumulated overnight – the source of "morning breath."

From here I head downstairs to the kitchen and it's time for coffee. While it's brewing, I read, write, or play online poker (a minor addiction) because I find that engaging my mind helps me to wake up. Writing and poker do this a bit more than reading – I can become drowsy reading, and to a lesser extent writing, but online poker is something I learned I can NOT do before sleeping because it really makes me alert, so I'll sometimes do it in the morning to get going.

In Closing

Writing this book has been a massive undertaking that has taken me a number of years — how many I've lost count of to be honest — more than 7. Many times, I thought I was ready and then realized I wasn't — there was more to figure out and tell you. Now, finally, I think and I hope that I have conveyed everything I have learned so that you can know what I know and sleep like I sleep.

Above all, I hope that we as a society worldwide can recognize and acknowledge that we have been waging a War On Sleep, and that it is time for that to end. We need to get back to proper rest cycles and better health so we can enjoy our lives, not just survive them. We were never intended for death by sleep disorder — we were meant to live well-rested enjoyable lives.

I sincerely hope that, starting tonight, using what I have shared your sleep will improve and continue to do so.

Acknowledgements

Special thanks to:

Dr. Noah Silverman for decades of friendship and collaboration on all things biohacking.

Dr. David Viscott and Dr. Gordon Livingston, may they both rest in peace, for timeless words of insight and inspiration. Two of the greatest psychiatrists to ever live – their brilliant words live on in their books and in my mind.

Jessica Grimwood – for copy editing and assistance of all kinds - I hope you actually read and use this book now that it's done!

Sleep Cycle (www.sleepcycle.com) – a great tool without which I would not have been able to gain and document most of my improvement in sleep this past decade. Almost certainly the greatest tool for sleep improvement on a mass scale ever created.

Dr. Nicholas Schenck – simply the best otolaryngologist anyone could ever ask for.

Special acknowledgment to the outstanding National Geographic video series Naked Science episodes Dead Tired and Sleepless in America. These are quite possibly the two best documentaries on present day sleep issues ever made and I highly recommend watching them for everyone reading this book. They were invaluable in providing me with information, resources and motivation.

About the Author

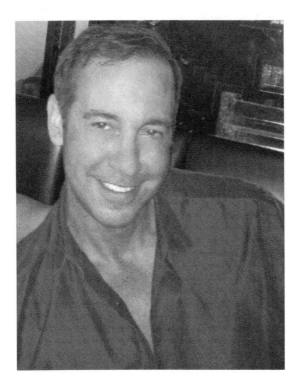

Michael Voss lives in Los Angeles, California where he is a computer scientist consulting on IT infrastructure and security issues. His interests include computer security research, biohacking (as applied to human performance, longevity and sleep), renewable energy, and poker. He speaks regularly to corporate audiences who want to help their employees and executives sleep better.

He can be reached at voss@waronsleep.com

Made in the USA
Middletown, DE
05 February 2022

60604554R00108